LEARNING THE HARD WAY

LEARNING THE HARD WAY

A CAREGIVER'S STRUGGLE WITH ALZHEIMER'S

Donna Grant Reilly

Copyright © 2018 by Donna Grant Reilly
All rights reserved.

ISBN-13: 978-1723364198
ISBN-10: 1723364193

Library of Congress Control Number: 2018908858
Donna Grant Reilly, Hanover, NH 03755

No part of this publication may be reproduced, distributed or transmitted in any form or by any means, including photocopying, recording, or other electronic or mechanical methods, without the prior written permission of the publisher, except in the case of brief quotations embodied in critical reviews and certain other noncommercial uses permitted by copyright law. For permission requests, write to meadowsidepress@gmail.com.

Ordering information available through Amazon.com.

Printed in the United States of America.

For Chuck

Also by Donna Grant Reilly

An American Proceeding:
Building the Grant House with Frank Lloyd Wright

CONTENTS

Foreword by Robert B. Santulli, M.D.   ix

Prelude   xiii

1	Is it Alzheimer's?	21
2.	How Will I Do This?	29
3	Change, For Better or Worse?	49
4	Struggling.	65
5	The Difficult Decision.	74
6	How Will I Know?	85
7	There Will be Doubts.	91
8	Transition.	97
9	Life in a Different Place.	108
10	Where Do I Fit In?	123
11	The Caregiver's Dilemma.	131
12	I Need You.	143
13	How to Avoid Learning the Hard Way.	152
14	A Long Illness.	164
15	All the Help We Can Get	169

Coda   174

Acknowledgements   177

FOREWORD

There are now more than 5.5 million people with Alzheimer's disease in the United States. As the population ages, it is predicted that the number of individuals with this progressive, incurable cognitive disorder will increase significantly. By the middle of this century, if no cure or prevention is found, there will be as many as three times the number of people with this deadly disorder.

Along with the growing number of people with Alzheimer's, there will be an ever-increasing number of individuals devoted to caring for them. Many are spouses, but there are also adult children, grandchildren, and others. Most caregivers are female.

While there are many good books written for the Alzheimer's caregiver, their focus is largely on how to care for a loved one with the illness, and much less on the emotional and psychological needs and reactions of the caregiver. Yet more than half of all Alzheimer's caregivers suffer significant emotional and psychological symptoms as a result of the enormous stress associated with this long and arduous undertaking.

For these reasons, *Learning the Hard Way: A Caregiver's Struggle with Alzheimer's* is an especially needed and most valuable contribution. It tells the heartbreaking story of Donna, the author, and Chuck, her beloved husband who has Alzheimer's disease. It begins with his diagnosis nearly a decade ago and continues through the present time. Chuck is now living in the dementia unit of their continuing care retirement community with significantly advanced disease. But, unlike many other books, this chronicle is told from the *caregiver's* perspective. With noteworthy candor, Donna describes the uncertainty, frustration, anger, guilt, sadness and other painful emotions she has felt, as well as the enduring closeness and love she has experienced as her husband's disease continues its inexorable course.

Donna and Chuck are fortunate enough to have the financial resources to be able to live in a marvelous continuing care retirement community with a wide array of support services for both of them and the comfortable and sensitive dementia care unit where Chuck now resides. Fortunately, they have been able to avoid many of the very difficult practical challenges faced by Alzheimer's families of more modest means. But this does not necessarily make the many agonizing thoughts and feelings experienced by Donna any easier. If anything, it highlights them.

A common misconception about Alzheimer's disease and its burdens on the caregiver is that once the individual is placed in a facility the stresses on the caregiver are dramatically reduced or even eliminated. This book makes it very clear that this is not the case. While some of the more difficult aspects of caring for someone at home are eliminated by placement, many other emotional and psychological challenges remain and new ones develop, such as the crushing feelings of guilt that nearly every caregiver faces after placing a loved one in a facility, no matter how necessary placement had become and no matter how fine the facility. And the feelings of sadness and loss are, if anything, made more acute by the physical separation that has now occurred. Nearly half of this book takes place after Chuck has made the transition to the dementia unit of their continuing care retirement community. Donna scrupulously recounts her many continuing reactions to the placement. This will be particularly valuable for those who may believe or hope that the burdens are substantially lessened or even eliminated by transfer to a care facility.

Most caregivers, particularly early in the course of the disease, long to have someone with whom they can discuss the many intense, unsettling, and painful thoughts and feelings which are aroused by having a loved one with Alzheimer's disease. Unfortunately, many are quite reluctant to reach out, for a variety of reasons. Even more than wanting concrete suggestions about how to manage the disorder, caregivers need to feel that they are not alone in experiencing the painful and often-bewildering sentiments engendered by this very difficult challenge. While there is no substitute for communicating directly with an understanding and sympathetic person who is, or has been, an Alzheimer's caregiver, the author's candor and expressiveness about her emotional and psychological responses throughout her husband's illness should reassure many that their own reactions are certainly not unique. Donna also shows us that, while the pain and sadness certainly continue, it is possible to gradually reach a degree of equanimity, and to have a meaningful life in spite of the disaster which is Alzheimer's. This is perhaps the most important message of this fine book.

Robert B. Santulli, MD
Hanover, New Hampshire
July 2018

PRELUDE

When my husband, Chuck, was diagnosed with Alzheimer's disease, it didn't come as a complete surprise. His grandmother and his mother had each developed severe dementia in their later years. His mother lived on the west coast, but we saw her often enough to observe that dementia was gaining the upper hand. This extremely vital woman was fading into only a faint suggestion of the intelligent, independent and strong-willed person she once had been.

    At roughly the same time, my father was developing dementia as well. By the time it was officially diagnosed, it had progressed considerably, due to the fact that my family had assumed Dad had Alzheimer's and nothing could be done about it. It turned out to be vascular dementia, the result of small strokes he'd apparently suffered in the recent past - events he probably never noticed. There isn't much difference between the two forms of dementia, but Alzheimer's is the more common of the two. The symptoms are virtually the same, and so is the rate of progression and the outcome. As far as treatments go, there are none that offer more than temporary relief. So, they had been right; nothing could have been done about it.

My father and I had always been close, maybe because I was the firstborn. Among the many things he taught me was how to listen to music. When I was a child, Dad had always played lots of classical music recordings, so I'd been exposed to it from an early age. One of his favorites was the Debussy String Quartet in G minor. I learned to like chamber music by listening to that recording. By the time I was an adult, it was one of my favorites, and I've always associated it with my father.

Dad's dementia continued to change him over the next few years until he no longer communicated much at all. He didn't recognize anyone but my mother and brother. I lived far away from my parents, so I didn't see them often. Now I can admit to myself that I hadn't made more of an effort to visit, because I couldn't bear to see Dad the way he'd become. I wish I'd had the courage to spend more time with him as he gradually faded away. I lost my chance to say goodbye to him. And I failed to understand how much Mother could have used more support in her role as Dad's caregiver.

She had been his only caregiver. My brother lived nearby, and helped where he could, but Mother took on the majority of Dad's daily care. She'd done it willingly, but it began to take its toll on her as the months went by and Dad's condition became steadily worse. Although I'd successfully managed to avoid seeing Dad, I knew Mother wanted me to come for a visit, and finally I did. The evening I arrived, after a dinner where Mother and I did all the talking, she suggested that I go into the study with Dad and listen to music.

"He always played music every night after dinner," she said. "He doesn't seem to be interested in it anymore; but maybe he'd like to listen with you."

As we entered the room, I asked him what he'd like to hear, but he indicated that he wanted me to choose. And so, of course, I chose the Debussy Quartet. We listened to it quietly, Dad smiling, and I remembering all of the things I associated with it. When it was over, the CD started to repeat. I looked over at Dad and said,

"Would you like to hear it again?"

He smiled at me and said nothing, so we heard it again. By the end of the second playing I thought we should listen to something else, but, I was unfamiliar with this machine, and I couldn't figure out how to turn it off. I asked Dad if he could tell me how to make it stop, but he just smiled. It was then I realized,

He's forgotten how to work the player. That's why he doesn't listen any more.

So we heard the quartet one more time. By this time, tears were streaming down my face; I was beginning to understand just what we had lost. My lively, intelligent, wonderful father was gone; someone who merely looked like him had taken his place. Now I was sobbing. I looked at Dad. He was looking at me and smiling, and I thought,

Is it possible that he knows? He may not be able to express it, but, somehow, I think he understands why I'm crying.

Chuck and I each watched a parent slowly disappear into dementia. I saw my mother's life almost destroyed by being a caregiver. So why, when I was confronted with the reality of Chuck's Alzheimer's, couldn't I remember how it had felt to see my father slowly changing and Chuck's mother turn into someone else? Why didn't I recall anything from those times that would have helped when my turn came? Why was I so selfishly preoccupied with my own grief that it never occurred to me to wonder about the wide range of emotions Mother must have been feeling. If I had just taken the time to sit with her and encourage her to tell me what her life as Dad's caregiver was like, it would have been good for each of us. She needed to talk about it and I needed to hear. But the opportunities passed, and I never had the benefit of her experience. Now I found myself walking the same path, with little or no understanding of which way to turn.

Are all of us who become Alzheimer's caregivers destined to endure the same struggle as those who experienced it before us? I don't think it has to be that way. But, if we don't want to keep playing out the same, sad scenarios, there's a lot we'll need to know. The best way to learn is by listening to those who have already been there and done that. They can tell us a lot.

I've written this book for everyone who's caring for a husband or wife with Alzheimer's. Because I'll be talking about my husband, I'll use the masculine pronoun, but it applies to both. I have been straightforward in my recital of our experiences, but Chuck is no longer at a place where this narrative would disturb him. As for the location and the characters, anyone who knows us can easily identify them. They are real people and places, but I've changed many of the names because I feel more comfortable doing so.

And, finally, this is not a "How To" manual; I don't think it's possible to write one. Each person's progression through Alzheimer's is unique to that individual, and there are certainly no perfect answers to all questions. I've tried to give you an honest account of what we've lived with during the last few years. Maybe, when you compare our experiences with yours, you'll be able to think about yours in a way that makes life a little more tolerable for both of you.

LEARNING THE HARD WAY

ONE

IS IT ALZHEIMER'S?

Chuck and I married in 1976, a second marriage for each of us. By that time, he'd already graduated from Dartmouth, spent four years on a destroyer in the Pacific as an officer in the U.S. Navy, received an M.B.A. from the Harvard Business School, and joined the ranks of those who manage other people's money. He was good at his chosen profession, and was at the height of his career when we married. He loved to read, mostly about history, economics and politics; he couldn't imagine beginning the day without reading the New York Times. He also liked to ski, play tennis and go for long hikes. He enjoyed a good, heated discussion – the more intense, the better. He had a wonderful sense of humor, and was able to see the funny side of almost any situation. We lived in New York's Greenwich Village, had many friends, and went to lots of parties and events, as well as concerts and lectures. I thought he was handsome, sexy, intelligent, kind, and thoughtful. He felt the same about me. We were very much in love.

Early in our relationship, Chuck told me his maternal grandmother had suffered from serious dementia near the end of her life. It appeared that his mother was now heading in the same direction, and he feared it would someday happen to him, since the genetic auspices were not favorable. I know he thought about it, particularly when his mother's condition was becoming steadily worse. But it's one thing to know you might be a candidate some time in the indeterminate future. It's quite another to believe it's really going to happen to you, especially when you're young and healthy. It certainly wasn't anything we talked about at length. We never gave a thought to what we might do if it became a reality someday. I wonder if anyone in that situation does.

I'm frequently asked,

"When did it start? When did you begin to think there might be some cognitive changes taking place in your husband?"

It's difficult to pinpoint any exact behavior that caught my attention. All of us who are aging think we're losing our memories when we can't think of a name or forget where we put something. How often have we walked into a room, only to wonder,

"Now, why did I come in here"?

In most cases, these occasional cognitive blips are part of the process of growing old, and rarely indicate any reason for alarm. But later, when I tried to remember any specific instances of uncharacteristic behavior in Chuck, I did recall some occasional memory lapses that had been merely annoying at the time, but not worrisome. In hindsight, they began to form a pattern that suggested something more complicated might have been going on.

During the 40 plus years of our marriage, we have travelled a great deal. We've been almost every place we wanted to visit – a few places more than once. After the first few trips, I'd started to do most of the arrangements; Chuck was happy not to deal with it, and I enjoyed doing the planning. After we both retired from our jobs, in 1990, we had more time to explore new places, and often we took two trips a year. We varied our itineraries. One year we did a self-driven barge trip down the Midi Canal in France, and followed it two months later with a two-week trip trekking through the foothills of Annapurna, in Nepal. It does seem now as though we were in a hurry to make up for lost time. There were so many things we wanted to do together, and we were reaching the age where we begin to grasp that time imposes limitations.

In the spring of 2008, we went on a delightful small-ship voyage. It began in Athens, passed through the Corinthian Canal into the Adriatic and on up the eastern shoreline. We stopped off at various countries along the way, such as Albania, Montenegro and Croatia, where we went ashore for sightseeing. The trip ended in Slovenia, where we stayed in Bled, on a beautiful lake by the same name, at the foot of the Julian Alps. We made some good friends on that trip, and thoroughly enjoyed one couple, Mary and George, in particular. We discovered we had a great deal in common with them and we often shared the same activities.

One morning, Mary announced that she was going to walk around the lake. Would we like to join her? It was a beautiful day and the ninety-minute walk appealed to us both. The path was wide enough for the three of us to walk together. We didn't encounter many people coming the opposite way, so we started off walking and talking. Shortly after we began, I noticed Chuck was lagging behind. We stopped several times, waiting for him to catch up, but he continued to drop back. At one point I asked him if he was feeling all right, and he assured me he was. I didn't really think he was sick. I was the only one who ever got sick on trips! Finally, I took him aside and said,

"Are you sure you're all right? Would you like to go back?"

"No," he said, "I'm fine. I just think you and Mary would like to talk. I'm perfectly happy back here." This was so unlike him that at first I thought he was joking.

"Oh, come on," I said, "You have to be in the conversation; we need your opinion. We aren't talking 'girl talk'".

Mary was concerned and asked me,

"Is he all right? He doesn't seem at all like himself."

I had to agree, but I dismissed it as something he and I could discuss later. By dinnertime he was fine, and back to his convivial, agreeable self again. The rest of the trip went by without incident.

But some time later, I recalled another example of surprising behavior on that trip. We had been transferred by coach from our hotel in Athens to the docks at Piraeus, and had immediately been ushered to our ship. We were just settling into our cabin when there was a knock on the door. There stood Alan, our tour leader, grinning widely and holding Chuck's passport. Chuck had left it in the coach when he got out, and Alan had discovered it. Usually, it was Chuck who worried about the passports, so this was a little disconcerting. We thanked Alan profusely, and we agreed it might be better if I carried both passports, just to be safe.

Around that time, there had been other, mildly unsettling events at home – isolated examples of discordant behavior. It had been Chuck's job to fill the two humidifiers in our house every winter evening; but, he left the water running in the bar sink all night on more than one occasion. No harm done, but still... Chuck had always made the coffee every morning, but now, sometimes, he forgot to put coffee in the basket or to add water to the coffeemaker.

On Friday mornings I attended a study group in town while Chuck played tennis nearby. Since we finished at about the same time, it seemed logical to drive in together and have him pick me up on his way home. But sometimes, after I had been waiting for thirty minutes, I knew he had forgotten me. As soon as I called him at home, he got back into the car and drove the twenty minutes back to town. He was sincerely apologetic, but I wasn't angry with him. I think I was starting to realize that all was not well. Our plan to save energy by using only one car was thoroughly dashed, though.

Over the next few years we took more trips, but now we depended on tour groups to do all the planning and arrangements. We still enjoyed going places, but I noticed that Chuck was becoming increasingly less willing to join group activities, aside from actual tour excursions. He preferred turning in for the night to staying around after dinner, being social.

I wondered if he should see a doctor – someone who could give an educated opinion about whether or not he might be in the first stages of cognitive decline. We discussed it; Chuck was reluctant to take that step, although he recognized there might be something wrong. I told our primary care doctor what we were considering and she heartily agreed that it was a good idea. She recommended a specialist, and soon we had an appointment.

Chuck had his first appointment with Dr. Foster, a psychiatrist, in August 2010. The doctor asked many questions and administered extensive cognitive tests. I read his notes about the visit later online. His conclusion was:

At this time, patient does not meet criteria for dementia, but shows some mild cognitive impairment.

This seemed oddly dismissive. "…some cognitive impairment?" I certainly thought it was more than that. I wondered about the difference between dementia and cognitive impairment, and what the criteria were for deciding, but I didn't ask.

However, Dr. Foster was concerned about Chuck's strong family history of dementia. He ordered an MRI of Chuck's brain and further neuropsychological testing before the next visit in six months. The MRI results showed:

Mild diffuse cerebral atrophy with slightly disproportionate medial temporal tissue loss and appearance consistent with Alzheimer's disease.

The date was September 15, 2010.

TWO

HOW WILL I DO THIS?

In the last ten or twelve years we've learned that an increasing number of Chuck's college classmates, or their spouses, are developing Alzheimer's. These are people who have been our friends for many years, whose anniversaries we attended and whose children we watched grow into adults with families of their own. We have seen the disease reach its slow but inevitable conclusion, and we've marked with concern the effects it has had on the spouse-become-caregiver.

When it was our turn, we were saddened, but not really surprised. Chuck has lived for many years with the knowledge that he might someday be a victim. Still, it was difficult now to accept it as fact. Almost two years went by before he could bring himself to break the news to his children. When he finally composed a letter to them, he showed remarkable courage and compassion for their feelings, knowing they would be horrified. But he asked them to regard the knowledge as confidential.

When Alzheimer's is diagnosed, the news is often received with varying degrees of acceptance. The reactions might range from outright denial to shock, sorrow, horror, and finally terror, by the victim as well as the spouse. Being aware that you might get Alzheimer's in the future, and being told you have it now, are two kinds of reality. Of course, we all know that someday we will die, but being told you have a disease for which there is no cure is altogether different. Knowing you are mortal provides cold comfort when you have been diagnosed with what amounts to a death sentence.

Chuck's children were understandably stunned, partly from disbelief. They hadn't spent a lot of time with their father in the last few years, so there had been little opportunity to experience his gradual decline. He seemed the same to them. I realized they had only a rudimentary knowledge of what Alzheimer's is and how it affects its victims. I've never known how much they thought about their own future health, but that might have been a factor as well. They are adults now; some have families, and they all have careers and lives of their own. But I think they hadn't yet reached that point when you realize that your parents won't live forever. Most of us don't, until we experience the loss.

During my discussions with Chuck at the time, I began to suspect that the diagnosis might not have entirely registered with him. He was perfectly amenable to conversations about the near future. It was he who initiated the decision to speed up the move to Wellman, a continuing care residential community where we had been on the waiting list for several years. But I could tell he preferred to avoid talking about Alzheimer's. As a result, I didn't press the issue, but it was always there under the surface. I now believe there might have been a part of him that understood the diagnosis well enough to know he didn't want to deal with it. If we didn't talk about it, maybe it wouldn't be true.

It's hard to understand, in the twenty-first century, why there is still so much about Alzheimer's that's a mystery to those who haven't experienced it in some way. Alzheimer's has been around for decades, but the name wasn't a part of popular usage until relatively recent times. I remember, as a child, hearing people talk about memory failure in an older person,

"Oh, don't pay any attention to him, he's just getting old and senile", or,

"Stay away from her; she acts a little funny."

Dementia was something people didn't talk about. If a member of your household was afflicted with it, people pitied you, but they gradually stopped coming to see you. Apparently it was assumed that, if you lost your memory, you were somehow rendered incapable of thinking about anything at all. You had suddenly lost all ability to control yourself, and might be capable of who-knows-what outrageous behavior.

What do you say to the family of a loved one with dementia? He doesn't seem to be ill, and he looks about the same. But he doesn't act the same anymore. Sometimes he's angry for no reason you can see. At other times he appears to be struggling - unable to communicate with anyone. The family isn't holding any sickbed vigils; but they seem to be mourning for someone who isn't dead. Today we know a lot more about the disease, but unfortunately, a surprising number of those old judgments linger on. Is it any wonder why someone with a diagnosis of Alzheimer's today might say to his family, "Don't tell anyone"?

Shortly after we began going for regular sessions with Dr. Foster, I scheduled a meeting with him, without Chuck, to try and learn what might be ahead for me. I asked him,

"What will be my role now? Can you give me some idea of what to expect?"

He spent a considerable amount of time describing the disease, and how it affects those who have it. It was interesting, and I appreciated the time he spent with me. But I began to have the feeling that I'd asked him questions he couldn't really answer. I had already read about most of what he told me, but I felt certain there must be more to it than that. I left his office with the uncomfortable suspicion that this was something I was going to have to manage all by myself.

At that point, I would have liked to talk with someone who had already been through what I was just beginning, but I had no idea of how to do that. I cannot exaggerate how alone I felt. Oh sure, I was ready to take on the job of caregiver. Hadn't we promised to take care of each other "...in sickness or in health, 'til death us do part"? I recalled how my mother had never questioned her role as Dad's caregiver. But, eventually, what had been a difficult job became a hellish nightmare. Much painful time had passed before we were finally able to convince her that he needed professional care.

I wish I'd asked Mother why she had thought it was necessary to bear this burden alone, rather than seek outside help -- at least part-time. I know their marriage was a long and loving one and they were especially close. She always said she couldn't bear to leave him with strangers, and I'm sure she really meant that. It's also probable, given my mother's fierce sense of loyalty, that she felt it was her duty to see him through to the end. As terrible as their lives had become, at least they were still together. My brother was a great comfort to her, and he devoted a lot of his time looking after both of them. But she had no one to talk to who might have been able to help her by sharing similar experiences. She didn't know anyone who could sympathize with her concerns and frustrations by saying to her,

"I understand what you're going through; I've been through it myself. Let's talk about it."

She was lonely at the end of her life; she missed Dad so much. I may have been close to my father, but no one was as close as he and Mother were. Now I can imagine what she must have been going through as she watched the love of her life gradually disappear, without entirely understanding how and why it was happening.

For the next few years, Chuck and I continued on a more-or-less even course. We continued to enjoy life in this house we loved so much. We took care of the gardens, stacked firewood for the fireplace and mowed the lawn. We had lots of parties and houseguests, because we enjoyed it. But it was gradually becoming more difficult to do these things. We were getting older, of course, but I also realized that Alzheimer's was beginning to make its presence known more frequently now. It could appear at awkward times.

One evening we'd invited good friends for dinner at our house. These couples happened to be neighbors, as well as friends, and we had dined together quite often. Talk at the table was lively, facilitated by good red wine, and everyone appeared to be having a fine time. As dinner was winding down, I realized that Chuck was becoming a little more argumentative than usual. His comments began to seem more vituperative than were called for. The friend to whom he was directing them was beginning to be uncomfortable, and so was I. The atmosphere was becoming a bit strained and, after a suitable interval, our guests said their goodbyes, thanked us, and left.

When we were alone, I asked Chuck,

"Why were you so hard on Tom? I think you hurt his feelings."

He seemed surprised by this, and appeared to be unaware that anything had been out of the ordinary. But he brushed it off as inconsequential, and never mentioned it again. I began to notice more instances of these outbreaks occasionally – not all were fueled by red wine – and many new examples of uncharacteristic behavior were appearing as well.

The following is from a journal I kept for a three-month period around that time. When I reread it a year or two later, I was surprised to discover what had been going on then, and how quickly the Alzheimer's was advancing. By this time, we had decided to move to Wellman, and we had sold our house.

March 1, 2014

Every evening now progresses more or less the same way. We begin with drinks in front of the fire, talking about events of the day or, more often, what we've been reading in the newspapers.

"Did you read Krugman's column this morning?"

"Yes, I thought his comments were right on the mark."

Things seem to be going well, and many nights it continues in that vein. But some nights we descend rapidly into confrontation mode where Chuck, pointing a finger at me, says,

"Well, maybe the problem is you. Think about it!"

Unless I can redirect these unpleasant conversations, we end by arguing in circles and, often, by screaming at each other. There never seems to be any real point to these arguments, and I know I shouldn't be entering into these excruciatingly painful exercises. Somehow, we still work our way through dinner. But he usually, in his words, "craps out" around 7:00 – 7:30, often electing to sleep downstairs in the guest room – without changing into pajamas, brushing teeth or taking his evening medication.

The next morning he seems fine. Sometimes he apologizes for his behavior, but often he doesn't remember why he was downstairs at all. We start all over again.

April 10

I'm not sure how much longer we can go on like this. It's clear we are getting on each other's nerves, but I don't see any way to escape from the depths to which we seem to have descended. He needs me to manage our day-to-day lives, make all the decisions, fix whatever goes wrong and keep life on a more or less even keel. He seems aware that I'm trying to do so, and often tells me,

"I can't tell you how grateful I am that you're taking care of everything."

But by the end of the day, he is resentful, insulting, argumentative, critical, and doesn't appear to like me very much. I try not to fight back; I know it's the Alzheimer's mandating his behavior. But recently he has started asking,

"Do you want a divorce?"

I don't think he means it, but apparently he believes it's something I want.

"No, Chuck, I certainly don't want a divorce. I love you and I want to stay married to you. Why do you ask me that? Do you want a divorce?"

His reply is always, "Well, it would be the solution to your problems, but, no, I don't."

I wonder if he realizes how dependent upon me he has become. He needs to know where I am at all times and, when he has forgotten where I've gone, he becomes accusatory when I return. His memory loss seems particularly acute in the last few weeks. He asks many times about something we've just discussed. At least I know better than to say,

You've already told me that four times now.

But that's what I'm thinking.

Right now we're going through a particularly difficult period as we approach the house sale closing on Monday. Chuck appears to understand that we are selling the house, but living here has been so special for us that I wonder why he hasn't questioned why we are selling it. We built this house twelve years ago, and we always expected it would be where we lived out the rest of our lives. I suppose it's entirely possible that he hasn't really grasped that the sale is happening. I've told him what will be taking place at the closing many times, but I fear he'll become confused and make it quite difficult. He insists on attending, although he wouldn't need to be there. He seems to feel things will go badly if he isn't there. He is quite capable of nodding in my direction and saying,

"Don't listen to her; she has no idea what she's talking about." Although I know he doesn't mean it, it isn't at all helpful. If we can get through the next two months – until June 25 – we'll be out of here and living at Wellman. In the meantime, I have so much to do and very little support. He wants to help, but isn't really able to. When I ask him to help me with something I think he's capable of doing, he either forgets what he was going to do, or does the opposite of what he started out to do. When I finally take over the job, I know he feels hurt and incompetent, but it has to be done.

His daughter is coming tomorrow for the weekend, and bringing her two dogs. Having someone else around always makes it easier. Chuck enjoys the dogs, and so does our dog, Ginny, so it will be a great diversion. If others are present, Chuck doesn't exhibit the same behavior patterns as he does when it's just the two of us. I'm looking forward to it.

I really hope living at Wellman will be better for both of us. We'll be around many old friends and will make new ones. Chuck and I see too much of each other right now, and we desperately need to expand our worlds. The pressure on me to get everything right and, at the same time, to be good natured and "fun" will be alleviated. I'll have more time to devote to my own interests, and I'm hoping Chuck will, too. Now, if we can just get through the time before we move, life should soon become a little brighter.

My greatest fear right now is that I'll become seriously ill or incapacitated in some way. I can't imagine how we would survive. We need to get to Wellman soon. How do other people manage this? Is it this way for everybody who is a caregiver?

April 26

The closing went well; Chuck seemed detached throughout the procedure, but it went off without a hitch. The buyers have generously agreed to let us stay in the house until June, when we move to Wellman. They seem genuinely fond of the house and I think they will take good care of it. I'm slowly becoming less fond of it; there are times I hate it, because I feel tied down here to a life I no longer enjoy. I'm beginning to understand what Mom was going through with Dad, but he was not combative. He was helpless and totally divorced from reality, but sweet and quiet during the years of his dementia. I miss him. I miss talking to him and sharing music with him.

I rarely have an opportunity to listen to music any more. Chuck, knowing how much I like it, frequently tells me that he wishes I would play music; but when I do, he complains that it sounds "screechy", and I end up turning it off. I've tried headphones, but I think he feels left out when I have them on. Recently, I played the Debussy Quartet. I hadn't listened to it for a long time, and I hoped it would relax me. Instead, I thought of my father and how quiet and uncomplaining he had been as his dementia progressed.

Chuck's son and his kids were here for a short time this week. I don't think they were prepared for what they discovered. This son has resisted accepting his father's condition; I suspect he doesn't really want to know more. The grandchildren were not prepared for what they saw, and I'm sorry they had to learn about their grandfather the way they did this week. But I know they are thoughtful and mentally flexible and, in time, will be able to process the information in their own way.

For a long time now I have dreaded evenings here. The paranoia and ugliness start immediately when we begin the "cocktail hour" at 5:00. I really don't think it's the alcohol entirely, although that is a catalyst. Chuck doesn't drink very much any more. He has one, hefty bourbon, with water and ice, and one glass of wine with dinner. But precisely at 5:00 I become The Enemy. It doesn't matter what I say, it's wrong. He might say,

"Anybody who thinks that is stupid," or, " That was a really dumb thing to say!" When I protest,

"You know, I don't like being called 'stupid'; it hurts me when you say that." He is likely to say,

" I didn't say that. Why do you accuse me of saying that when I didn't say it?"

It's impossible to carry on a conversation with him, but he bemoans the fact that "we can't communicate any more". The evening frequently ends with Chuck storming off to bed in the downstairs guest room around 7:30 – 8:00. But by the next morning, he's forgotten that any of it ever took place. I've been told this behavior toward the end of the day is typical of Alzheimer's; it's called "Sundowning". I'd do almost anything to avoid it.

At the same time, I do believe the deterioration has increased in the last month. He forgets things he has always done from long habit – simple things, such as knowing where we keep kitchen equipment, or how to make coffee. He doesn't remember if he fed the dog, shortly after he has done so.

One of the more problematic situations has become his desire to cook on the outdoor grille. He had been doing this very well for many years, but has gradually lost the skill and versatility he used to have. But he insists that he cook dinner (or lunch) on the grille, and often the results are far from perfect. I plan for three or four meals a week that he can grille, but we often eat meat that is either undercooked or overcooked. He asks my opinion about how long he should cook everything, but usually disagrees with what I suggest. I also worry about the propane, and whether or not he has turned it off. I often creep out to the back deck after he is asleep to make sure everything is secure. Thankfully, there will be no more outdoor grilling at Wellman!

May is almost here, and then it's less than two months before we move.

May 3

Tonight we had a small altercation about which direction was west. It's pointless to argue, because when Chuck is confronted with the truth, he says he didn't say that. It reminds me so strongly of the summer, many years ago, when his mother was staying with us on eastern Long Island for a week. Helen was exhibiting strong signs of dementia at the time. She and I were there alone during the week; Chuck was still working in New York and joining us on weekends. Helen, firmly settled on the California coast, could never accept the fact that Long

Island is situated almost east/west along the NY coast, not north/south. It was impossible to convince her otherwise. One evening, as the two of us were enjoying a before-dinner glass of wine, the subject came up again. I stood up and said,

"Come on, Helen, let's get in the car. I want to show you something."

She agreed and we drove across the bridge to the barrier beach where the sun was beginning to set. We parked, got out of the car and walked along the beach.

"Okay," I said. "In what direction does the sun set?"

She laughed and said, "In the west."

Triumphantly, I said to her, pointing to the setting sun, "So what direction is that?"

Again she laughed, and said, "Well, I guess it is west."

Since that time, I've outgrown that annoying need to be right. I expect Helen was going through the same stage of dementia then that her son is now. It was as pointless to insist that she admit which direction was west as it is to expect that Chuck will remember what I told him fifteen minutes ago.

I'm learning a great deal more about myself these days, not always knowledge I'm happy to accept, but now that I'm in my 80's, it's about time I do. I'm also discovering that a certain amount of ingenuity is useful when one is required to solve problems for which there often seem to be no answers. Mostly, these days, I try to concentrate on all of the delightful things I remember about the man I married more than 40 years ago. But, more and more, it's becoming harder for me to remember that he's the same man.

May 12

    For all of our married life, we celebrated what we loved about each other. I thought he was wonderful, brilliant and fun to be with, and he felt the same about me. We had such great times together, sharing information, gossip, thoughts, and ideas. We felt comfortable with each other and reveled in the fact that we'd never had this kind of relationship before. I could say anything to him about what I was feeling, thinking, wondering. He was a strong mentor and gave me encouraging support at a time when I needed my confidence restored to its old levels. He taught me so much I needed to know about myself, about the world and my place in it. I will always be grateful to him for that. I think I did a lot for him, as well. I taught him that everything doesn't have to be a contest. Some of the best times are those when we just relax and enjoy what we see and feel around us. And I helped him learn what it's like to trust somebody. I would never have written my first book without his encouragement, help and support. When it was published, he was my greatest promoter. We've had a great life together for the last 40+ years. Not perfect, but very close to perfect.

But that has all changed. This terrible disease has taken away the best parts of the man I love and left us with a lonely, sad and anguished relationship. Most days begin well; we joke and laugh and work around the fact that his memory is mostly gone. His hearing is steadily failing to the point where he doesn't hear a lot of what I say. He guesses about the part he didn't hear, and the result is often disastrous. But by 5:00 PM, he continues to change into a totally different person. He's argumentative, insulting, angry, and the memory loss is greatly exaggerated. I have come to dread the "cocktail hour" because it's the breakdown of all communication between us.

What is it about this disease that affects each person's brain the way it does? I have known others who suffered from Alzheimer's, who gradually became quieter, more withdrawn and dependent upon others. In our case, it has produced some harsh sides of his personality I never knew existed. Indeed, he seems to be following closely in the footsteps of his mother, who managed to alienate everyone around her as her dementia progressed.

I can no longer venture an opinion about something without being accused of being "shallow, stupid or not thinking". It seems that all his pent-up frustrations, fears and terrors are being taken out on me. We no longer have a supportive relationship. Either he doesn't want to get involved in decision-making or is fearful of trying, so I now make all decisions and hope for the best. In most cases, I think I'm quite capable, but I'm constantly afraid that he will suddenly question my right to do so, because he understands so little of what goes on day to day. But maybe that's only a reflection of my own insecurities about assuming an unfamiliar role.

I really don't know what to do next. At times, I fear the best recourse is for me to completely give in to his demands, and resign myself to a situation where I accept his criticisms without argument. I wonder if I'm capable of it. I suppose I can force myself, but at what cost? I need to be strong; I'm all he has. I know he realizes that, and often expresses his gratitude for my "tolerating" him; but there's a part of him that is fighting it. I don't know if I'm strong enough to keep on walking down this treacherous path.

May 21
I understand I have lost my husband to a terrible disease. He may look the same, and sometimes show glimmers of the man he once was, but the

old Chuck is gone. Knowing that and dealing with it are two different things. I know he can't help his behavior, and I understand I must make allowances for much of what I don't like. Tonight we ended with a screaming, ugly fight. I can always see them coming. It's almost as if he starts baiting me, waiting for me to explode. I'm being tested to see how much I will take before I break. And, although I know it's counterproductive, sometimes I do break. I wish I could talk to someone who understands, but I can't imagine unloading my troubles onto someone else. I don't feel I can burden his family with it, and I'm reticent to talk about it with friends. Tomorrow he will have forgotten everything that happened tonight, but sooner or later I know it will happen all over again. If we could just get away from each other for a while it might not be so awful. I'm concentrating so hard on the move to Wellman; it's my only hope.

    This is the part of Alzheimer's they don't tell you about. We only read stories about how a loved one gradually drifted away quietly until he or she ended up in a long-term care facility and stayed there until the end. You seldom read anything about accusatory, hateful behavior from a loved one who's fighting every step of the way and lashing out at the one who loves him the most, and is always there to take it.

THREE

CHANGE, FOR BETTER OR WORSE?

Our moving preparations were no different than anyone else's. We suffered through all of the questions about what to take with us, what to sell or give away, and what to throw out. Moving from a big house to a three-room apartment involves making momentous decisions, none of them easy. It's probably not necessary to mention that Chuck wasn't much help during this period. In the best of times, those decisions would probably have been mine, anyway, and now he wasn't the slightest bit interested in them. We had a giant garage sale, and then I called the Man With a Truck Who Will Take Anything. Somehow we got everything packed and the movers came and took it all away.

The physical move to Wellman was even worse than I'd thought it would be. Moving is never fun, especially when one is downsizing. It went reasonably well, but I vowed we would never do it again. When we began the moving process, I thought I'd figured out just how much to take with us. But the day we moved in – when I'd filled up all the storage space in the apartment, and discovered there were still twelve unpacked cartons lined up in the hall outside – I knew the worst was far from over. I worried that Chuck would be disoriented, but he concentrated on making sure that Ginny, our dog, was comfortable, and he seemed to be fine.

Within a few days, however, he began to say he missed our house and ask why we had moved. Eventually, he became more vocal, saying,

"I hate it here! I hate everything about it. I wish we hadn't moved." I would think to myself,

> Well, you knew we were going to move here and you were very much in favor of it. I did all of it myself, and you were no help at all. I didn't want to leave our beautiful house, either. The only reason we did was because of you.

I understood that everything seemed wrong to him. I sympathized with him, saying,

"Oh, I know it's been really rough. I've been so busy I haven't spent much time with you, but it will soon be back to normal and things will be better."

After a while, there were more distressing signs of change in his personality. This wonderful, level headed husband, who had always been the one to calm me down when I got carried away, began to complain about little things he didn't like. He missed our large bathroom. He didn't like his shower, and he didn't like the way I had decorated our apartment.

"Why can't we have an apartment that looks like everybody else's? Ours is ugly."

> I've knocked myself out to get this apartment in shape. I think it looks great, and so does everybody else who's seen it. You used to tell me I was good at making our home look attractive. Just stop complaining all the time!

He didn't want me to go out for long periods of time, and he was often angry with me when I returned home. I knew from experience he would be perfectly all right at home by himself. Many people with Alzheimer's often wander off and become lost. Fortunately, Chuck was not a wanderer, and usually just took a nap when I went out.

One day, a Wellman friend with a dog asked me if Ginny and I would like to join her for a walk. I told Chuck where we were going and about how long I thought we'd be gone, and we set off. Apparently, I wasn't thinking clearly, because I decided I didn't need to take my phone. About an hour into the walk I realized it was going to take longer than I'd thought, so I was relieved when we started back. We were a long way from home and, when I returned, I had been gone for almost two hours. I knew something was wrong as soon as I came through the door. Chuck was furious and looked it.

"Where have you been?" he said, shaking with anger.

I tried to explain and apologize for my long absence, but he was too upset.

"I finally called the police when you didn't come back. I didn't know where you were."

"Oh dear," I said, "What did the police say they would do?"

"While I was talking to them, I saw you out the window, coming back, so I told them you were back and to never mind."

I was doubtful this would be the end of it and, sure enough, I soon had a call from the Wellman nursing station. The nurse told me they had received word from the police regarding the phone call from Chuck, and was everything all right? I assured her all was fine and described the situation. When I apologized for the fuss we'd caused, she explained that, when Wellman residents call the police, the call is immediately reported to the nursing station, which then follows up by contacting the resident. I was impressed, thanked her profusely, and assured her we were back to normal. I should have known there would be more to come. A few minutes later there was a call from the receptionist downstairs,

"There's a policeman here to see you."

I quickly told her the story, asked her to tell him everything had been sorted out, and to thank him for me, but I didn't feel as if I should leave Chuck at this point. Later, when things had calmed down a bit, I said,

"I'm sorry I was so late; I didn't realize how far we were going to walk. But you knew where I was going." He replied,

"I forgot."

From then on, I always left a note stuck to the mirror in our entrance hall, saying where I was going and when I would be back. And I always took my phone. I think it was then that I began to fully grasp how far along the Alzheimer's had progressed. It was apparent that Chuck was no longer able to maintain much, if any, short-term memory. I still wonder how he was able to locate a telephone number for the police.

Although I had guessed the move would be traumatic for him, I wasn't prepared for just how disoriented he became. Everything was new and strange, he couldn't find anything, and didn't know where to look. I showed him, over and over, where everything was stored, but I should have understood that he couldn't retain that knowledge. At times, the sound of him opening and closing drawers, trying to find something, nearly drove me crazy.

> What are you looking for? If I hear another drawer banging shut I'm going to start screaming. I can't stand this!

But it wasn't his fault; he was frantic when he couldn't find what he wanted. I made labels for the cupboards and drawers, hoping it would help. It did help a little, but not entirely. He began blaming me when things went wrong. We argued a lot, mostly about things that weren't terribly important. I knew arguing accomplished nothing, but I seemed to get trapped into it. Most terrible of all was when I finally understood that his capacity for absorbing and comprehending information had gone. He would often say,

"Why can't we talk anymore? Why can't we just sit down and discuss our problems?"

That's what we'd always done; talking things out and finally arriving at a solution that worked for us both. Now we would sit down to talk, but the discussions never went anywhere. They went around and around, covering the same ground over and over again, until I burst into tears and ran out of the room, frustrated over what I knew would never be any different.

It wasn't long before I began trying to avoid these "conversations".

> I'm beginning to feel like Scheherazade, trying to think up things to talk about every night. Sometimes I'm just too tired to make the effort, but I don't like the silences when neither of us says anything. It doesn't seem to matter anyway; whatever we talk about goes nowhere.

We had been living at Wellman for about a year when I started to notice another change in Chuck. He was playing tennis year-round, about two or three times a week, with the same group of friends. He was an accomplished player and was enthusiastic about the game. We had come to Wellman with two cars, so we could go our separate ways during the day. This arrangement worked well for a time, but he began calling me from the tennis courts, saying,

"I can't find my car keys; I guess they're lost. Could you bring me the spare set?"

In truth, they weren't lost; often they were in a coat pocket, or sometimes they were still in the ignition. I made the 15-minute trip more than once, only to learn that his keys had miraculously appeared by the time I got there. He knew the way to the tennis courts and back, but if he had to drive somewhere else, he would ask me how to get there, even if he had driven there many times. The day he left the keys in the ignition, with the engine running, in our parking lot, I wondered if it might be time for him to stop driving. There were other signs as well. He had always been an excellent and careful driver, but now he would turn and talk to Ginny in the back seat while we were driving on the highway. Soon, he wouldn't drive anywhere without me in the seat next to him, but he always wanted to drive.

    I thought he would never give up driving without a hard fight, but I was wrong. At my suggestion, the Wellman health center gave him a written drivers' cognizance and reaction test. I took the test, too, because I thought he would be less suspicious if we both did it. I was with him when he took his test, so I wasn't surprised when we learned the results. He had done so poorly, he was advised to stop driving right away. Fortunately I had passed the test, so we still had transportation. He received the verdict with incredulous disbelief, but he accepted the fact that he would no longer be behind the wheel of a car, and he hasn't driven since. There were times in the next few months when it was clear he had forgotten the entire episode, and I would need to remind him that he wasn't driving anymore. We gave his car to his youngest son, and I became the designated driver.

My husband has always been the life of any party; he was friendly, funny, loved to joke, and he carried on good conversations. One of the things that I'd found attractive about Chuck in the first place was his ability to converse easily with both men and women. It may sound surprising now, but that was a rare quality fifty years ago. He read a great deal, and devoured the newspapers every morning. His favorite subjects were economics, world events, politics and sports. But now he began to show less interest in reading, and I soon realized he was reading the newspapers over and over again. At the same time, he became impatient with the evening news on television. He would say,

"Everybody talks too fast; I can't understand what they're saying. This isn't news. I want to hear news!"

and he would storm out of the room, only to return in a few minutes and repeat the same scenario.

> Why do you get so worked up about this?
> You've always enjoyed the evening news
> hour. Why can't you just sit back and
> watch it the way you used to? If you
> think I'm going to get up and follow you
> out, you're wrong. I'm going to watch
> the news.

He was right about everyone talking too fast; that seems to be the norm these days. But his insistence that there was "no news" puzzled me. After talking with him at great length, and gently questioning him about the way he viewed the news, I finally realized that his brain could no longer process what it was reading or hearing. He couldn't comprehend the concept of an "in-depth" news story; therefore, it no longer seemed like news to him. Although this development was clear to me, it wasn't to him. I decided there was little to be gained by trying to explain it to him. He would only deny it.

Some of the residents who knew Chuck before we moved to Wellman began to ask me if he was all right. Several told me,

"He doesn't seem very happy anymore. He doesn't smile and laugh the way he used to."

He spent more and more time on the screened porch of our apartment. He seemed quite content to sit there looking at the newspaper, watching the activity in the parking lot below, and talking to Ginny, curled up on her bed beside him.

Oh, yes. Ginny. We moved into Wellman knowing our dog would need to be on a leash any time she was outside our apartment. A ten-year-old chocolate Labradoodle, she was smart, wonderfully shaggy, remarkably obedient, and good company. We loved her dearly, and she returned our affection in her own way. She seemed to adapt quite well to the leash, and all was going well until Chuck began removing it as soon as he reached the bench in the courtyard where he liked to sit. Ginny was content to mostly lie at his feet and watch the birds and the people, but she got up occasionally when approached by someone who wanted to pet her.

The complaints began soon, however. It appeared there were some residents who had appointed themselves Dog Monitors, and who enthusiastically embraced the job of reporting any violators of the rules. Apparently, Chuck had been "spoken to" on one or more occasions, but had cheerfully shrugged off any admonitions, and Ginny continued unrestrained. When I found out about it, I tried to explain to Chuck why he needed to keep her leashed. I used all the standard reasons: some people were afraid of dogs, and there were numerous fragile, elderly people who were afraid of being jumped on. The leash laws were necessary to protect all residents. He just said,

"She doesn't need to be on a leash. She's a well-behaved dog and she obeys me perfectly."

Sometimes, he even promised he wouldn't let her run loose anymore, and I think he really meant it at the time. But he continued to take her leash off as soon as he got outside, and the complaints continued in earnest.

> There they go, walking through the parking lot below, and Chuck has Ginny on the leash. He promised me he would leave it on this time. Maybe he's really going to do it. Please, please, let him keep her on the leash!

But when they came into view on the return trip, Ginny was running loose, ahead of him, and I wanted to cry.

> Oh, no! He promised. But of course he doesn't remember that, and he never will. It's just never going to happen.

I finally got a call from a member of the staff, insisting that I make Chuck keep the leash on the dog. When I asked him how he expected me to do that, he said,

"Well, you'll have to make him understand or he won't be allowed to walk the dog anymore."

It wasn't that Chuck was blatantly breaking the rules to defy anyone. He just didn't remember that he wasn't being compliant. He honestly believed Ginny didn't need to be on a leash, so he saw no need to leave it on.

In the next few months, I had several serious discussions with the staff member, trying to explain that my husband had Alzheimer's, and how the disease affects people. I began doing all of the dog walking, but then, of course, we argued about why I wasn't allowing him to do it. That plan worked as long as I was home to take her out, but it was destined to be a failure from the very beginning. The occasional medical appointment, meeting, or anything else that took me away for a while, was the one, unavoidable weak link. As soon as I walked out the door, I knew Chuck would take Ginny outside again, without a leash. I felt helpless and depressed by the entire situation, knowing full well what the inevitable conclusion might be.

Gradually, over the next few months, I noticed that Ginny's behavior was changing. Our normally laid-back dog had become jumpy and skittish around other dogs and was less willing to let people pet her. I thought it was just because she was getting old, but I began walking her in places that were less populated. She had always been a dainty eater, but now there were times she refused to eat much at all. Concerned, I took her to her veterinarian, but she passed her examination and was considered to be in good health. We were puzzled by her behavior, but there didn't seem to be anything wrong with her.

Finally, we started to realize that, when either of us walked into a room where she was resting or sleeping, she silently got up and left. I remembered she had always been uncomfortable with any quarrels or tension between the two of us. We had rarely raised our voices to each other in the past, but that had changed as the Alzheimer's progressed. Also, after we moved, we no longer had a big house with many rooms, and there was no dog door where Ginny could come and go outside whenever she liked. Now, there was no way she could get away from us if she wanted to. I began to understand what was wrong with Ginny. She had lived a happy, carefree life with us since she'd been a young puppy; we taught her what kind of behavior we expected and we gave her a lot of love. When Chuck's Alzheimer's symptoms began to be more pronounced, I'm sure there were subtle changes in our behavior, with more arguments and strained silences. Dogs are remarkably sensitive to our moods, probably because they have a lot of time to observe us, but also because they are dependent on us. They may not always know what we're saying, but they read our facial expressions, tones of voice and gestures. I understand now how much we were changing. I had been so wrapped up in my own worries that I had failed to notice that it was we who were making our dog sick and unhappy.

I finally got the call I had been dreading from our intractable staff member, who told me,

"If you can't stop Chuck from taking Ginny out without a leash, we'll have to ask you to get rid of her."

I knew I would never be able to make Chuck understand, and I knew that losing Ginny would be unbearable. But there was never any possibility of another option.

I set about finding a solution I could live with. I couldn't bear the thought of taking her to a shelter, but If I could find someone who really wanted a dog, and whom I could trust to give her a good home, it would be easier to go through with it. Remarkably, the solution appeared almost right away. I found Ginny a home with good friends who had just lost their dog. They were happy to take her. When I returned home after delivering Ginny to her new home, I was prepared for Chuck to be upset. He clearly didn't understand what had happened or why. He asked me many times, "Why did you get rid of her? Didn't you want her anymore?" At one point he asked me, "Did you put her down?"

> Oh, Chuck, I'll never make you realize how awful this has been for me. I loved that dog so much, and you did, too. It was one of the hardest things I've ever had to do. I'll miss her and I know you will too, but you'll never understand why she had to go.

Ginny's been gone for two years now, and I hear she's doing well. She is happy with her new home and has returned to being the dog she used to be. Her new owners love her dearly. It took an enormous toll on both of us, and I still shed a few tears when I talk about her. But, even if giving her away made us sad, it released a lot of pressure that had been building for some time. Now that I no longer had to worry about Ginny, I could relax a little and be more tolerant of our situation. These days, Chuck sometimes says to me,

"Do you think we should get another dog?"
And I reply,
"I don't think so."
He doesn't pursue the subject.

FOUR

STRUGGLING

A few months after we moved in, Chuck began to get used to his new environment. He was starting to accept that we lived at Wellman now, and it would be our permanent home. Occasionally he grumbled about it, but he no longer complained so much. He appeared to have established a routine he could live with. I was happy to have left all the worries, work and stress of the move behind us. But I recognized that it was time for me to come up with a way of life that would work for both of us.

No longer frantic to get us physically settled, I tried to reestablish as many of our former routines as I could within the parameters now available – the cocktail hour, the evening news, the Sunday brunch and an occasional lunch out. Chuck's weekly tennis games fit easily into our new schedule, and went on without the slightest disruption. Everything about our environment was new, and the move to Wellman was making our lives considerably less complicated. But, in trying to get us back to a normal routine, I had failed to take into account the one thing that hadn't changed. Alzheimer's had followed us to Wellman, and was definitely here to stay.

I felt very much alone for a while. I had friends and acquaintances here, some who were aware of our situation, but I really didn't want to burden them with my problems. We went to dinner with many of the residents, and met lots of them who became friends. But Chuck grew less fond of going to the dining room unless we sat with people he knew well. His behavior at dinner was fine. He always started out with jokes and laughter; but before long he was asking the same questions over and over. When he was asked about his former career, or questions about events in his past, I was startled to realize that he cheerfully made up the answers as he went along. His hearing wasn't good, and the noise in the dining room reverberated through his hearing aid, making him extremely uncomfortable. If someone at the table spoke too softly, he strained to hear them. I think it embarrassed him to keep asking, "What?" Finally, he simply fell silent while everyone else conversed around him; he had tired of trying to keep up.

After awhile, very few people asked us to dinner. Occasionally, we tried eating at a table for two, but we often ended up arguing. Chuck's hearing made it impossible for me to speak to him in a lowered voice, so I'm sure everyone near us was privy to our conversations. Or at least I thought they were.

> I hate this! I feel certain that everyone can hear us or at least see that we are arguing. Yes, I'm embarrassed. You bet I am! I'm sure everyone is feeling sorry for us, and they're probably talking about us as well. Why can't I just accept this behavior? I know it's the Alzheimer's, and I hate myself for being embarrassed. Why do I even care what other people think?

Soon, by mutual agreement, I started going down to the dining room and bringing our dinner back to the apartment, or I cooked it myself. I had observed many others doing the same, and it became the perfect solution for us. We could now watch the news before dinner and eat when we were ready. Chuck was much calmer, and I didn't have to indulge in my paranoid speculations about what others were thinking.

But the arguments and the fighting continued. I knew it was the wrong thing to do, that it only exacerbated our problems, but I let myself become involved in these sessions. And they never ended pleasantly. Finally one Friday evening, we were standing in the kitchen and Chuck was yelling insults at me,

"Maybe you should think about whose fault it is! Have you ever thought it might be your fault? Or are you too stupid to understand?" I grabbed his arm hard and said,

"Stop yelling at me! I don't like being yelled at. Everybody walking past our door can hear everything you say!"

The combination of my grabbing his arm and scolding him was too much for him. He gave me a hard shove across the kitchen and I slammed into the counter. I looked at him in disbelief. Anger was contorting his face, and I suddenly understood that there had been a dramatic shift in the progress of this disease. We were in new and unfamiliar territory now.

> Good lord, what is happening here? I don't know this man. He's never done anything like this before. He's a lot stronger than I am, and he is really angry with me. I should never have lost my temper. I know he'd never hurt me, but what if he does lose control some day? What would I do? I don't know how to handle this.

I succeeded in calming him down, and the rest of the evening was uneventful. But I knew I would have to find an answer to that question. What would I do?

The next morning I called the Nurses Station, because I didn't know anyone else to call. This was a weekend, and the clinic for independent living residents was closed. I described my concern to the nurse in charge, and she quickly assured me that they are capable of handling any situation, with whatever means seem necessary at the time. She asked me if I thought I was in any danger, and I assured her I was not. I was greatly relieved to hear her reassurances, and I felt more secure, knowing someone was there in case I needed them. Monday morning, I had a call from the Head of Nursing, who asked, again, if I was worried about my safety. She reinforced what I had been told the night before. I remembered that this was why we had moved to Wellman.

If I could start this caregiving job all over again, but this time with a better understanding of what was happening to both of us, would it make any difference? Would I do it any other way? Would it be any easier? Will I always need to learn everything by trial and error?

I understand now that I had gradually been moving from a relatively tranquil life, with a husband who was my partner in every respect, to a life that had lost all semblance of any kind of order. Most of us expect to have some degree of normalcy in our day-to-day lives. We make plans for the future, work around various bumps in the road, spend time with our friends and family, and take part in activities we enjoy. In other words, we usually have a pretty good idea of what is coming next each day. Living with Alzheimer's has destroyed any semblance of that kind of existence. There is no normal; order has turned to chaos. It will drive you crazy if you let it.

I had undervalued the importance of talking to others about my problems. In doing so, I was missing out on one of the best resources available to me – the benefit of other caregivers' experiences. At first, of course, we were newcomers and, outside of a few people we already knew, we had little information about our new neighbors. We had yet to learn who they were, what kind of lives they had lived, and how they had adapted to life at Wellman. When I met people in the halls, they had often asked,

"How are things going for you and Chuck?" I'd always answered,

"Oh, just fine, thank you."

But things weren't fine. There were times I wanted to scream, but there was no place to do it without being overheard. On more than one occasion, I left our apartment hoping that no one could tell I'd been crying. One or two women, whom I didn't know well, told me their husbands had been in Harris, the dementia care unit at Wellman. They'd said,

"Any time you want to come and talk, just let me know."

But I wasn't ready to do that just yet. Two of my friends here at Wellman had been genuinely interested in how we were adjusting to our new situation. When they'd asked me,

"Is everything okay?"

I'd finally understood that they were asking because they really wanted to know, and so one day I said,

"Well, it could be better."

It was to those two friends I eventually turned when things started to get really rough. I was beginning to fear I might not be able to handle our situation by myself, and I had no idea what to do about it. Each of them had suggested that I might like to meet for coffee, and talk about what was on my mind. So I began to share my concerns and frustrations with them. It wasn't easy at first; I was hesitant to unload my troubles onto someone else, but they encouraged me to talk. And it all came pouring out – along with a lot of tears – all the doubts and frustrations that were keeping me awake at night. My friends couldn't provide solutions, but they could listen, and they did. I would leave these meetings exhausted and drained, but I felt the load was lighter for a while, just by having shared it.

Eventually, though, I felt guilty about taking up so much of their time. I feared they would soon tire of these painful revelations, but wouldn't want to tell me.

> I'm sure they're thinking, "Oh, dear. Here comes Donna again. I know I should listen to her, but I've heard it all so many times." I don't want to lose my dearest friends. I feel so much better after talking with them, but they must be sick of hearing my troubles.

I was immensely grateful for what they were willing to do for me, but I wanted our friendships to go back to the way they were. I wanted to spend my time with them talking about things that interested us, relaxing together, laughing and enjoying each other. There was a caregivers group at Wellman that met on a regular basis. I didn't want to join it, because we knew some of the people who attended it; some had been Chuck's college classmates. This probably sounds ridiculous, but I was determined not to undermine his dignity by sharing accounts of his ugly behavior with the group. Although he was difficult to live with, I was fiercely protective of him.

As I became more acquainted with our medical care provider, Dr. Gordon, and the rest of the medical community at Wellman, I realized that they were a source of support I hadn't thought much about. I began seeking out Ingrid, a community support professional at Wellman, and spending an occasional half-hour in her office. She's an energetic, upbeat individual who impressed me by her no-nonsense approach to problems. Instead of saying,

"Oh, honey, I'm so sorry this is happening to you!" she was more likely to say,

"Well, gee. Nobody needs to put up with that kind of stuff!"

What's more, she had suggestions about things I could try that might make our lives a little more peaceful. Dr. Gordon gave me as much of her time as I needed. She was sympathetic, supportive and supplied me with straightforward answers to the questions I asked. And gradually, I was able to feel confident that I understood the path I had to take, and where it was leading. How wonderful it was to know there were people who were willing to make it as easy for me as possible.

FIVE

THE DIFFICULT DECISION

We took another trip in April 2016, a barge trip on the Loire Canal in France. Chuck now depended on me to do everything. I was happy to, knowing he was no longer capable of taking any responsibility at all. When we arrived in Paris, we had time for a luncheon meeting with my college roommate who lives there. Chuck is fond of her, and I always look forward to seeing her. We had an extremely enjoyable reunion, comparing notes on what our children were up to and commiserating about current political outrages. Although, Chuck didn't really take part in the conversation, he seemed to be enjoying it. Afterwards, we had our photos taken with the Eiffel Tower in the background to prove we'd actually been in Paris.

    The first morning on the barge, Chuck awoke in a panic, shouting,

"There are people out there in our yard doing things! I've got to get out there and make them go away!"

We were docked along the canal, and there were men doing maintenance work there. It was all I could do to restrain him from rushing out the door of the cabin in his pajamas, to investigate. I finally succeeded in reminding him where we were, and the rest of the trip continued without further disorientation.

In spite of its rocky start, we both thoroughly enjoyed that trip. There were twenty-four passengers on the boat, and everyone got along splendidly, even though half of them spoke only French. Chuck seemed relaxed and was able to converse reasonably well with those who spoke English. I think it may have been because we were meeting everyone for the first time; he wasn't expected to remember names and faces. Several of our new acquaintances were able to grasp that he had some cognitive impairment, but they treated him with compassion and respect. It couldn't have been a better situation. I was also pleased that my careful planning had paid off; I had finally learned what was necessary to make traveling with Chuck an enjoyable experience. I needed to arrange every leg of the trip to insure he would be comfortable and worry-free. That meant doing my best to plan for all the unforeseen screw-ups I could imagine. It worked beautifully, and I had a brief respite from worrying if our lives could ever be peaceful again.

We'd had good luck renting vacation houses each summer after our move to Wellman, so this year we rented a tiny cabin on a lake in New Hampshire's Lake District for the last week in August. It was a pleasant drive, about an hour and a half away, and it turned out to be a delightful place. The owners lived nearby and were friendly, helpful and considerate of our privacy. I had brought enough food and supplies with us so we didn't have to rush out to shop right away. First, and of paramount importance, I established that the nearby convenience store carried the New York Times, and then we unpacked and settled in to our temporary home.

The week went well. We took it easy and didn't try to do too much in the way of exploration. We had our own private beach, where we spent time almost every day. Chuck wasn't interested in going into the water, which seemed strange. He used to be a fine swimmer and always enjoyed being either in the water or on it, in a boat. Now he seemed content to just bask in the sun and watch what was happening on the lake. That suited me just fine. We spent a lot of time talking about what a nice day it was and watching the sun slowly move across the sky. Each observation was made as if he was noticing it for the first time; in reality, he was just making the same discovery over and over again. His brain was no longer able to collect and store those observations for future use.

We went out for a few meals, but mostly we just stayed put. I had worried about the gas grille outside the cabin, thinking it might revive some of the conflicts about grilling we'd experienced in the past. Fortunately, Chuck seemed oblivious to it and the subject never came up. There was no television or radio, but I had my laptop and phone, and we had the newspaper. There was just the right amount of civilization. Chuck seemed quite content with this solitary life we were leading – just the two of us, alone together. Our conversations were still difficult, but we didn't fight. We often just sat in silence. At first I was uncomfortable with the long moments of silence, but gradually I realized they were not painful for Chuck. So I tried to do as he did, and enjoy the quiet times. But, pleasant as it was for a week, I'm not sure I could have made it through another one.

One evening, the owners invited us to dinner at their house, and we enjoyed getting acquainted with them. We discovered we had many things in common and several shared interests. It was a nice break for me, and I thought Chuck was enjoying it, too. He had retained a surprising amount of social awareness, which he could tap into on occasion. But, as the meal was coming to an end, I sensed he was becoming restless, and it wasn't long before he politely thanked our hosts and began his leave-taking. I'm sure they understood, even though the dessert course was about to be served; I had mentioned to them earlier that he was having some difficulties with his memory. When the week was over, we packed up and left, vowing to come back the next summer.

So far, it seemed we could take an occasional vacation, providing the arrangements beforehand could be worked out satisfactorily. A summer rental was very little trouble to arrange and, now that we had a place we liked, I quickly made the necessary plans to rent it again for the following August.

An out-of-country trip was a little more difficult, time-consuming and expensive to pull off. Nevertheless, remembering how much Chuck had enjoyed the barge trip in France, I got online in January and booked a similar barge trip for the following April. I also booked two business class seats on Air France. By this time, it was quite clear that Chuck would be miserable traveling overseas in coach. I had tried the pricier airline fare for the previous trip to France and found it solved a lot of major problems. First of all, we had priority going through security and boarding the plane. We had full use of the airline lounges and, best of all, we had seats where we could actually stretch out and sleep. Expensive as it was, it made the difference between a reasonably pleasant trip and a spectacularly bad one. I vowed I would never again do it any other way, as long as it was at all possible.

The winter of 2016-2017 was a difficult one. The weather wasn't bad for New Hampshire, not a lot of snow or bitterly cold temperatures. But it just seemed as if the gray, sunless days were endless; it was dark when we got up in the morning and dark again by the time we went to bed. Chuck had given up skiing several years before, and had no interest in walking outside. The walks were always cleared of snow, but the benches were still piled high. It was too cold to sit for very long anyway.

At least he still played tennis two or three times a week at the college's enclosed tennis facility. The guys he played with were wonderful about getting him to the courts and back. A number of them lived at Wellman, so most of the time I didn't have to drive him. I was extremely pleased with the ninety-minute breaks it gave me during that time, and I will always be grateful for their thoughtfulness. Chuck still played a good game of tennis. He had played for years, enjoyed it thoroughly, and always worked at making his game better. He was no longer quite as quick to get to the net for a drop shot, and I suspect he had no idea what the score was. But he knew what his opponent's weaknesses were, and took advantage of them whenever he could. He still had a mean crosscourt backhand!

In fact, one of the things that saved us from going off the deep end that winter was a subscription to a TV tennis channel. What a lifesaver it was; non-stop tennis 24/7! It didn't matter who was playing or when. We saw tournaments in places where one would never imagine there were tennis courts. Chuck no longer had much of an attention span, and he was anything but a dedicated television watcher, but he spent an amazing amount of time watching tennis. As a result, even though I once played the game, I began to learn more about tennis than I'd thought there was to know. We watched players no one had ever heard of before turn into tournament champions as the months went by. It was the best thing we could have done at the time. Chuck loved to follow tennis, and he understood what was going on. I usually taped the matches, so we could watch them later, without the frequent commercial breaks that made Chuck impatient. It didn't matter if he didn't hear what the commentators were saying; he didn't need the sound. There was no plot, and nothing complicated to understand. There was no need to remember what had already happened because it was all there on the scoreboard.

The winter seemed to go on forever. We didn't have a dog to walk anymore, which meant we could sleep a little later in the morning. There were no more mad dashes into blizzards or ice storms because the dog needed to go out, but we both missed Ginny. Chuck talked about her sometimes, always asking why I had sent her away. He showed no interest in hearing about where she had gone and how she was doing. He didn't remember what had happened or why. I saw no reason to go over it again. It didn't really matter what I said; it would eventually leave his mind forever.

He found it harder to be alone now. He would protest when I told him I needed to go to a meeting, even if it was going to be here in the same building.

"I don't see why you have to go. Just tell them you aren't going."

"Well I can't do that. They're depending on me to be there."

> I'm going to this meeting because I want
> to and because I need a break from you.
> If I don't get away from here occasionally
> I think I will die of cabin fever!

I continued to go to meetings, attending as few as I could get by with, often leaving before they'd finished. I worried about staying beyond the time I'd told Chuck I'd be home; I didn't know what would happen if I were to arrive home much later.

There were many classical music concerts at Wellman, and I always made it a point to attend. The concerts featured skilled and accomplished musicians who performed at a professional level. We knew we were fortunate to have them come and play for us. The performances were well attended, and enthusiastically received. Chuck has never been a fan of classical music, and had no intention of starting now. But he had always encouraged me to attend concerts, because he knew how much I enjoyed them.

One evening I told him there was going to be a concert that night, and I planned to go. He protested, as he usually did, but I assured him I would be gone for only a little over an hour. Our concerts were always programmed with no intermissions. And, out of respect for the aging bladders in the audience, they rarely lasted past 8:30. This time, however, he wasn't content with my answer. With genuine fear in his voice he said,

"I don't want you to go. Please don't go!"

I asked if he wanted to come with me, knowing full well that he didn't. Of course he said no.

> I know you don't want me to go, because you don't like it when I leave you. But I've

been looking forward to this all week. I need to get away and do something I enjoy for a change. If I stay home, we'll just sit around saying the same things over and over. Eventually we'll have a nasty fight, because I'll resent not being able to go to the concert.

I went anyway, feeling guilty, mean and despicable. As soon as it was over, I hurried back to the apartment, not knowing what I would find when I got there. Chuck was in bed, asleep. When I woke him to tell him I was home, he said,

"Oh, how was it? Did you have a good time?"

But now I started to understand that he was feeling not just insecurity when I left, but real fear. I can only guess what was running through his mind,

"Is she leaving for good this time? What if she doesn't come back? What will I do if she leaves me forever?"

There was a part of him that knew my life was difficult; he often told me how much he depended on me. At those times he told me over and over,

"I love you and I need you."

It finally reached the point where I couldn't stay very long in the bathroom before Chuck would knock on the door and call out,

"Are you all right?"

I believe he was truly alarmed that something might have happened to me. I think the fear had been there for a longer time than I realized. I wanted so badly to think of a way I could help this man I loved more than anyone in the world. I guess that was when I finally let myself think about what my mind had been pushing to the background for a long time. There was a way I could help him. Was I strong enough to make it happen?

SIX

HOW WILL I KNOW?

In February I had a long talk with Dr. Gordon. She had been extremely supportive during the entire time we'd been at Wellman. She always urged me to come and see her whenever things got tough. She had raised the idea of Harris, Wellman's dementia care unit, before. I'd asked her to tell me how I would know when it was time for Chuck to go, because it seemed so difficult for anyone to determine. There is no one answer that applies to everyone. She said,

"If the time comes when you feel you can't take care of him by yourself anymore, let me know and we'll talk about it."

Occasional home care was out of the question; Chuck had steadfastly refused it. I decided to continue on the present course for now. It seemed to me that his dementia had been steadily getting worse for several months, but I had no real basis by which to judge this – only my own observations.

By early April I thought it might be time for him to have another medical evaluation; it had been about six months since he'd last had one. I asked Dr. Gordon if she could do some more cognitive testing, and she agreed that it would be a good idea. He tested well physically. He was still in reasonably good shape, except for a noticeable weight gain and his ongoing hearing loss. The cognitive tests weren't so encouraging, though. There are 30 segments to the test, all designed to measure one's ability to retain information. In the past he had scored mostly around 20 or 25 out of 30; this time he scored only 13. Apparently I hadn't been imagining the decline in his memory.

Chuck's hearing has not been good for several years, largely the result of his being a gunnery officer in the U.S. Navy during the Korean War. Apparently, the Navy hadn't understood what duty inside a gun emplacement, without sound-blocking headphones, was doing to human hearing. Eventually, he had consulted an audiologist and began wearing hearing aids, but the loss was becoming significantly more pronounced. He now wears only one of his hearing aids, because he finds that wearing both is more than he can tolerate. He refuses to accept the explanation that he needs two, and that his brain would soon adjust to them. But a single hearing aid is better than not hearing anything at all, and so we've settled on one.

Several recent scientific studies have indicated a possible connection between hearing loss and dementia. People with significant hearing loss appear to develop dementia sooner than those with normal hearing. The temporal lobe, the part of the human brain that processes hearing, also plays a vital part in memory retention. Shrinkage in the temporal lobe is one of the few indications of Alzheimer's that can be measured as the disease progresses. It's probably not unreasonable to believe that there might be a connection.

In Chuck's case, I think the reverse is true as well; Alzheimer's is affecting his hearing. Because he can't grasp the reasoning behind what it would take to make his hearing better, he declines to accept the opportunities to do so. Therefore, his ability to process sounds functions at a much lower level. Poor hearing drastically affects his ability to communicate with others and, as a result, he is angry and frustrated a great deal of the time. Imagine how it must feel to see people around you talking animatedly when you can't hear most of what they say and you can't fill in the gaps. You do as he has done; you just quit trying and tune out. How terribly lonely he must feel at times. But maybe he has lost the ability to assess it that way.

The atmosphere at home was becoming so strained that I often woke in the morning in tears. We no longer had much to say to each other; we existed in an atmosphere of uncomfortable silence. The thought of facing another day like all the others was almost more than I could bear. We had reached a point where I couldn't leave the apartment in the evening without Chuck pleading with me to stay. I had remained determined through all of this that I wouldn't let it break me, but I could tell I was losing this battle.

Occasionally, I'd think ahead to the additional care that Chuck would eventually need as Alzheimer's continued to take control of him. I knew that, sooner or later, he would become unsteady on his feet and too heavy for me to support. I wouldn't be able to lift him if he fell and hurt himself. We haven't reached that place yet, but when I am forced to look ahead to what will most assuredly begin to occur some day, I can't avoid what's inevitable. The time will come when he won't remember how to control his bodily functions, and that will embarrass him. He'll forget how to feed himself, and he won't remember how to get dressed. And someday, he won't remember who I am and why I am there.

I thought a lot about what would happen if I got sick, or broke my leg and had to be hospitalized. What would become of Chuck? The staff assured me, whatever happened, they would take care of him. I knew it was true, but it didn't make me feel any better. One day, in Dr. Gordon's office, I recited a substantial list of things that were worrying me. She listened carefully, and then she said,

"Donna, I think it's time for Chuck to go to Harris."

I knew she was right. I needed to take that giant step, and I could no longer come up with any reasons why it wasn't the right decision. If there was a chance that Chuck and I could regain at least some of what had once been a loving and trusting relationship by moving him to Harris, then I knew I had to take that chance. So I agreed to the move, and we discussed what would happen next. Then I went back to the apartment and sent emails to his kids, telling them what was going to happen.

The reactions were varied, from shocked surprise to incredulity or sad acknowledgement. The medical staff had offered to arrange a telephone conference call with the family, so we set it up for the coming week. During the call, with Chuck's daughter and both his son's on the line, there were many questions – they had obviously given it a lot of thought. The staff was honest and forthcoming. They explained as much about Alzheimer's as they could, and answered questions patiently and concisely. There were doubts expressed about the necessity for making the transition,

"Does he really need to go now?" and "Wouldn't the transition hasten his death?"

The kids had questions about where their father would be living and who would be caring for him. All were responded to with thoughtful and detailed information. After Dr. Gordon explained how the transition would take place, and described the process of adaptation to the new environment, Chuck's son asked,

"Has there ever been anyone who never adapted?"

She replied,

"Not in the twelve years that I've been here."

The call lasted until every last question had been asked and every opinion expressed. I was extremely impressed with the entire session. I felt immense admiration and gratitude for the professionals who had taken the time to try and make this momentous step as acceptable as possible to Chuck's family. It was an important contribution to making the transition a little easier for them to think about and the reason for it a little less complicated.

The next morning, I began the task of cancelling the trip to France and the lease on the cabin by the lake.

SEVEN
_____

THERE WILL BE DOUBTS

We know our spouse has Alzheimer's, and there's presently no cure for it. Much has been written about it and we've learned, according to demographic studies, that there will be many more cases in the years to come. Considerable research is being conducted to find out what causes it, how it can be treated and, ultimately, how it can be prevented. If you are a caregiver for someone with Alzheimer's, you probably already know all this. You also know that your job is hard, emotionally and physically. You've devoted your life to the care of someone whose life is deteriorating as you watch. Do you let yourself think about what might happen next? What do you worry about when you lie awake at night?

"If I don't take care of hIm, who will?"
"We can't afford to hire extra help."

"He's my husband. It's my job to take care of him."

"I couldn't bear the idea of putting him into a 'home'."

"No one understands him the way I do."

"He would be miserable without me."

These are most certainly things to worry about. But try thinking about it this way. If your spouse had been diagnosed with cancer, you'd be caring for him, but you would also be getting help from medical personnel, therapists, and others trained for the job. If his condition required hospitalization, would you worry about him missing you or being lonely? You might, but you'd understand he needed specialized care. When his condition became worse and the end was near, wouldn't you rather know he was receiving all the care he needed to make his final days painless and peaceful? Shouldn't this apply to Alzheimer's as well?

But, even admitting that all of the above is true, there's still likely to be an unspoken concern haunting you. You worry that others will be thinking,

"How can she do that to her husband? It's just cruel and selfish of her to send him away like that! She's just dumping him."

You worry about what others might think, because this has occurred to you, too. But it's also entirely possible that other people are thinking,

"Well, she's finally decided to do what she should have done a long time ago. I don't know how she's been able to stand it all this time!"

What's important now, is that you decide what is right for both of you. That's what matters most.

When we think of dementia care, many of us are painfully aware of what we've read about the lack of decent healthcare facilities for those who suffer from Alzheimer's or dementia of any kind. There are too many news stories these days about people with dementia who have been mistaken for intruders or suspected of criminal behavior. The results of some of these "mistakes" have been disastrous and incomprehensible. My generation can look back on tales about "homes" for those who had become "senile" in their old age. If an aged relative without a surviving spouse became difficult to care for, it was usually assumed that the unmarried daughter or sister (maiden aunt) would be the caregiver. If there wasn't anyone who answered that description, and no money to pay an outsider, about the only other recourse was The Old Folk's Home. Often, there wasn't much difference between that and the Poor House in many communities. As the years went by, there were smaller birth rates, and grown children found it necessary to leave home for better opportunities elsewhere. At the same time, a burgeoning population of elderly people was living longer, but with dementia, and other maladies that accompany old age, as the cost. As a result, the need for better care soon became critical.

Eventually, retirement communities began to spring up across the country in places where seniors liked to retire, places with milder climates and good entertainment choices. With these communities came health care facilities for the elderly, ideally staffed with medical personnel who had embraced the practice of Geriatric Medicine (but mostly not, due to an insufficiency of practitioners in this field). By 2010 there were about 1,900 continuing care residential communities in the United States, with more on the way.

But, in many cases, there are varying opinions about what constitutes good health care. Years ago, Chuck, his sister and I tried to find a suitable facility for their mother, who was living in California. Her dementia had become steadily worse, to the point where she needed a great deal of care. We looked at several senior homes with dementia care units, but most of those we saw seemed too institutional. They were clean, and probably the staff was adequate, but the ambiance felt cold and impersonal. We couldn't imagine leaving her there to live out the rest of her life. Fortunately, thanks to her doctor, we were able to find a private home with comfortable accommodations and attractive surroundings. The couple that owned it was licensed by the state to care for elderly people in their home. They were kind and welcoming, and they provided a loving and friendly place for her to live – for the ten years until her death.

One of the hardest things about being the caregiver for a husband with Alzheimer's is forgetting sometimes that he has the disease. That's not as strange as it sounds. During the early stages of Alzheimer's, people often don't exhibit many of the characteristics associated with it. Even after the disease has progressed for quite a while, it's difficult for anyone outside the family, who only see the person occasionally in social situations, to believe there is anything amiss. There were many times when, darkly humorous as it may seem, I would forget that Chuck couldn't remember. In the days after he was scheduled to go to Harris, there had been bright spots in the day, when he seemed briefly like the lovable and fun-loving husband I knew so well. At those times, I had wondered,

> Have I made the right decision? Maybe I should hold off for a while.

But those flashes of sunlight didn't last, and we soon returned to long silences or angry accusations. By the time the date had arrived, I knew it was the right choice, and I tried to keep my focus on the time ahead.

I'm fully aware that there are many people who don't have the range of choices that we had available to us. Not everyone has a good dementia care facility near them and, thanks to the sorry state of health care insurance in this country right now, many don't have the financial resources required to even consider that choice. Although hiring professional caregivers is a viable option, the ability to choose that option will also cost more that many people can afford. I believe, however, that most of the things I'm sharing with you apply in almost any situation. All caregivers have one thing in common. We are caring for someone we love who has Alzheimer's. We want to find out how to do that job in a way that will make the situation as comfortable as possible for both of us in the best way we can.

EIGHT

TRANSITION

Very few Alzheimer's patients volunteer to leave home for better care. But it's not because they fear the place where they'll be going; they may not even know it exists. If your husband could tell you why he'd never want to go, it might sound something like this. Moving from independent living to a dementia care facility represents to him the end of his ability to perform an important and useful role in society. Some part of him knows he's lost the skills necessary to participate and compete in the world today. He is no longer able to enjoy things the way he did before. He's confused, scared, and very much afraid of what will happen to him now. Finally, no matter how unpleasant living at home has become, it's still the port in the storm he knows, with it's own reassuring routines. And, of course, he doesn't want to leave you - you're his only remaining anchor to security.

Now we had to start thinking about how we would manage the transition. The medical staff and I knew Chuck would never agree to enter Harris, even on a gradual basis. It would have to happen all at once, and a great deal of careful planning would need to be done ahead of time. His two sons wanted to be present for the transition. They lived in different states, so it was necessary to find a time when each could drive here on the same morning. It would have to be done on a weekday, so all the relevant staff members could be here. Dr. Gordon and Harris Director, Erica, would play a key role in the proceeding, and my friend, Alice, had volunteered to help in whatever way she could. Despite the number of participants involved, we found a date that worked for everyone, Wednesday, April 12, and we began working on the details.

    I had put together a list of furniture and personal belongings, such as pictures and art objects Chuck was fond of. These would be moved to his room at Harris, so he'd be surrounded by things he recognized. The facilities staff agreed to hold off coming for them until I could get him out of the apartment. I could imagine his concern, trying to puzzle out why his favorite chair was being carried out of our apartment by complete strangers. We arranged a physical therapy session for him with the therapist he was accustomed to seeing. The plan could go into effect as soon as he'd left for the appointment. His sons tried to time their arrival close to 11:30, the time his PT session would be ending. The boys planned to meet us in the reception area, and take him off to lunch. While they were gone, Alice and I would finish setting up his room and, by the time everyone returned from lunch, the transition team would be waiting for us there. I planned to meet Chuck and his sons when they returned from lunch and escort them to Harris. I hadn't yet worked out how I would explain this.

As the date approached for the transition, I was apprehensive – no, I was terrified – that something would go wrong. I was feeling a multitude of emotions about what was going to take place: anxiety, guilt, remorse, grief, and relief. Yes, relief. I had known for a long time that I was doing only a passable job of caring for Chuck. Even though I'd understood what Alzheimer's meant, and had thought I was prepared for what was ahead, I had never really known what to expect. I doubt if anyone ever anticipates at the beginning what life will be like as Alzheimer's progresses, unless they've had prior experience. Would it have been any easier if we'd known, ahead of time, that the stress level would become enormous and would never let up? Or was it better that we didn't know, and just found out as we went along? Unfortunately, that is what most of us do. That's why we desperately need someone we can talk to while it can still make a difference. If I hadn't had any outlet for that stress, I think my brain would have been close to shutting down.

    Two days before the moving date, I got a call from Erica, telling me an outbreak of Influenza A had occurred in the Health Center. Everyone there was in quarantine. That meant nobody in and nobody out; the transition would have to be postponed. Fortunately, I was able to get the message to everyone involved. We went back to life as usual while we waited for the quarantine to be lifted. For me, the postponement was similar to arriving at the hospital, only to be told that the surgery you'd been dreading had been rescheduled for next week. Now I'd have to start building up my courage all over again. Thankfully, Chuck was completely unaware that any of this was taking place. Two weeks later a new date of April 26 was set and we began again.

    Everything went as planned. Alice helped coordinate the move with the staff and, miraculously, we got the room ready in time. It looked as if it had always been there by the time the group came back from lunch. When they returned, I greeted them, asking if they'd had a good time, and other small pleasantries. I knew I'd have to think of some way to get them to Harris without raising suspicion. Chuck was aware that I occasionally did some work on an art project with Harris residents, so, as nonchalantly as I could, I said,

"Say, before we go any farther, I want all of you to come and see where I work some of the time."

I led them down the hall and into Harris. The rest was not so easy.

Dr. Gordon and Erica were waiting for us when we got to Chuck's new room, but now came the hardest part of all. It was time to break the news to him, and explain that he would be living here from now on. It took him a few minutes to deal with the appearance of familiar furniture and artwork in new surroundings. Looking confused and anxious, he said,

"What's going on? Why is my chair here?" Dr. Gordon immediately took over the role as bad news bearer.

"This is where you're going to be living now, Chuck," she explained. "Donna can't take care of you anymore in the way you need, but we will make sure that you are well taken care of here."

His reaction was every bit as horrible as I'd feared it would be. It took a while for him to process the information he was being given but, when he did, he was incredulous.

"We don't need to move here," he said. "We can afford to stay in the apartment."

Dr. Gordon explained again, and he finally began to grasp the situation. He lashed out at me because he assumed I was responsible and, in a way, he was right. He looked at me, anger distorting his features, and said,

"Do you want me to be here?"

All I could do was nod my head. I didn't trust myself to speak. At one point, I thought he'd shouted at me, "Get out!"

But, when I stood up to leave, he came running after me. Soon the whole group ended up in the hall outside his room. Chuck was shouting at me, I was miserable, and everyone else hovered around the two of us, trying to help. At this point, one of the nurses joined us and started talking to him in a way that he began to respond to.

"Listen, Chuck, I know you're angry, you're really pissed. But sometimes we say things when we're angry that we don't mean, and we're sorry later."

As she continued talking to him, she motioned for me to leave, which I quickly did. I learned later that, shortly after I left, Chuck told his sons to leave. I'm sure they were happy to do so, since they'd been visibly shaken by the entire scene. They hadn't been totally convinced that he'd needed to make this transition, and probably his reaction had only reinforced that conviction. As I burst into the reception area, I was sobbing so hard that I was finding it hard to breathe. Dear Alice was there to get me back to my apartment. She understood that I needed and wanted to be alone for now.

Some time later, both Erica and Dr. Gordon called to see how I was doing. Other than feeling that I had been the victim of a hit-and-run accident, I was managing reasonably well. Erica told me, that after everyone left, Chuck sat down with Julie, the nurse, and started to calm down. He began exploring his new surroundings, and talking with Susan, an old friend from our pre-Wellman days, who was now his neighbor across the hall. Erica said that, even though the episode had been so painful for all of us, Chuck appeared to have forgotten it entirely. When his son called me later that evening, I told him what Erica had said and he was incredulous.

"Really?" he exclaimed.

Incredulous as it may have seemed, we had just been given an example of the unpredictability of the Alzheimer's world.

Erica had told both of Chuck's sons that they were welcome to call her at any time to ask how their father was doing. One or the other called her every day for a while, but she said they didn't seem convinced when she told them he was doing quite well. She sent them photos of Chuck she took during the day, playing with a visiting dog, talking with other residents. After a couple of weeks, the calls ceased.

I was advised to stay away for at least ten days before going back to visit Chuck. My presence so early in the process would only have triggered more confusion and anxiety on his part. Now, alone in our apartment, I went over what had just happened and why. And, for the first time, I started to think about the time ahead.

> We've gone through this painful process, because we must gradually build trust between Chuck and the staff. Once that trust has been established he will begin to understand that Harris is where he lives now, and they are his caregivers now, not me. Once he accepts that, he'll eventually feel safe, protected, and confident that his needs will be met. Right now, that's hard to believe, because the whole thing has been so dreadful for both of us; but I desperately want it to work. Please, please let it work!

But it wasn't going to happen quickly. This was a major life-change Chuck was suddenly being asked to accept. I don't think I was entirely ready, either, to acknowledge that my role as caregiver was now essentially over. After all the doubts and wringing-of-hands, could transition to Harris really be that easy?

Two weeks after that tumultuous day in April, I went to visit him and we had lunch together in the dining area. He had been told I was coming, but kept forgetting. So, when I walked in and greeted him, he was speechless. I gave him a big bear hug that lasted for a long time.

"I thought you were gone for good," he said.

He was so happy to see me, and I was completely choked up. Lunch went well; we sat with Susan, and Erica joined us for a while. After lunch we sat in the living room and talked until it was time for me to leave. That didn't go so well. Chuck, of course, thought I had come to take him "home" to the apartment. We had to go over the whole business again, trying to reassure him that he would be all right at Harris. Chuck has never been one to accept what others say without question, and that part of him was still alive and well. He put up a good fight, but Erica was able to distract him. I left hurriedly.

Subsequent visits continued to go well. I went to see him once a day, usually after lunch. We went out for a walk when the weather allowed. We mostly talked about the weather and people who passed by, Chuck making the same statements over and over. I guess I'd thought that would change once he got to Harris. I'd assumed the difficult conversations had somehow always been connected in his mind with me being his caregiver, the person who managed his daily life. Now that others were assuming that role, we might be able to have normal conversations again. Apparently that was not going to happen – we still talked about the weather almost exclusively. Any topics I thought might be of interest to him drifted away without taking hold. He seemed to have no hesitation about going back to Harris after our walks. It was only when he realized I would be leaving him there that the difficulty arose. The fact that he was expected to remain there wasn't his primary objection; he just didn't want me to leave.

When word got around that Chuck had moved to Harris, everyone we knew expressed condolences in some way. I was touched and moved by their response but, at the same time, their sympathy seemed oddly inappropriate. He hadn't died! He was still with us, alive and well, just in a different place where he would be cared for by people who knew what they were doing. I could see him whenever I wanted, and I eagerly embraced the idea that our times together would be much more enjoyable. I know those who cared about us were sympathetic, knowing we would no longer be living together. I also knew they were aware of at least some of the stress that had been destroying us. It was important to me that everyone understand what was good about this major step we had taken. I wanted them to see the positive side of our situation. Recently, I met a neighbor, who said,

"How is your husband doing? Is he better now?"

"Yes," I said, "we both are.

NINE

LIFE IN A DIFFERENT PLACE

The first time people visit Harris, they're seldom prepared for what they find there. It's located on the ground floor at Wellman, in a separate wing next to the main entrance. Once you step inside, you think you're in another world. The walls are painted soft colors, the lighting is warm, and there are paintings and prints on every wall. Music is playing softly, and there's the soothing sound of trickling water coming from a large aquarium. There are planters full of greenery in many shapes and sizes, and attractive chairs and loveseats. You could easily imagine relaxing here.

The residents' rooms line both sides of the main corridor. There are a total of fifteen rooms; they are quite spacious and each has a half-bath and a large double window. If some of the doors are open, you can see that each room has been lovingly furnished with items familiar and meaningful to each resident. Furniture, paintings, keepsakes and potted plants make each space look comfortable and personal. Each room has a photo of the resident on the wall next to the door, with a short biography underneath.

At the center of the facility, the corridor opens onto a large area with spacious windows on both sides, where the sun streams in all day. This space has a living room on one side, with many comfortable chairs and couches, filled bookcases, lamps, plenty of tables for coffee cups, and lots of flowers and plants. There's a small alcove with a television set and comfortable seating. Next to the living room is a piano, with chairs arranged around it in a semi-circle. That's where concerts and sing-along sessions, or other leader-led activities are held each day.

The opposite side of the big space contains the kitchen and the dining area, which is located in a solarium. There are tables for either six or four, arranged to facilitate easy access for wheelchairs and walkers. The tables are covered in tablecloths and set with flatware and cloth napkins. There is usually a small bouquet of flowers on each table. The staff serves all meals, with a menu offering several choices for each meal posted on a nearby wall. A corridor off this area leads to more residents' rooms, a shower room and a whirlpool bath.

Outside the living room is one of the most charming garden spaces you'll find anywhere. It's quite spacious, with winding walks, benches for sitting, and arbors covered with robust climbing hydrangea. There's a terrace with an awning, which is the site of afternoon tea and cookies in summer. The landscaping includes lovely flowering trees, bushes to attract the birds, and flowers in many colors, available for picking. It's well populated with chipmunks and squirrels, whose antics are the source of much interest. It's a delightful place to sit on a fine day, listening to the birds chirping and the bees humming. I call it "The Cloister", because it's completely protected by majestic hedges, and it's wonderfully quiet and peaceful there.

The residents of Harris have varied personalities and talents. Chuck appears to have found a regular group with whom he can talk, join for meals and share activities. The residents are sometimes willing to engage in joking and conversation – and sometimes not. Almost all of them participate to some degree in the many activities that take place every day. Whether it's listening to someone play the piano, playing trivia games, tossing a balloon around, or simply engaging in quiet reflection while listening to a harpist, each joins in or simply enjoys watching.

Some of the activities require more engagement, such as painting, drawing, and baking. Others are more directed toward physical fitness, such as exercises to strengthen the arms and legs. The staff is gentle with them, always encouraging and never scolding. Their wants and needs are taken care of, and their idiosyncrasies indulged whenever possible. Some of the residents are single-purposed, with personal issues often preoccupying them to the point where they no longer have the desire to be social. Others are occasionally withdrawn and silent, lost in some world known only to them. But many haven't yet lost their sense of humor or their ability to kindle a spark in others. They are all still able to take pleasure in the small things that make the day brighter.

I'm convinced that Harris is a good place for Chuck to live, but I didn't just drop him off there and go back to my previous life, without a backward look. It was a terrible wrench for both of us, and the transition to life there has sometimes been difficult for us as well.

Understandably, it takes a while to accomplish a successful transition to a dementia care facility, but it does happen. It's difficult for a wife, who has done such a long caregiver stint, to turn over the job to professionals who will be doing it from now on. It's a transition for her, too, and it takes a while to get used to the idea. Now it's up to her to figure out the best way to continue her relationship with her husband, within the facility's framework. What works for some, fails miserably for others.

Eventually I fell into a regular visiting schedule that, most of the time, now feels comfortable for both of us. In our case, it means going for a walk around the Wellman campus in good weather, attending a Wellman event together, or staying at Harris for a meal. Maybe we'll attend an athletic event at the college or, if I'm feeling courageous, we'll go out to lunch. Routine is an invaluable tool in building a successful transition to a dementia facility. Anything that is pleasant, and occurs on a regular basis, is comforting to someone with Alzheimer's. That's the way the day is structured at Harris, and so I try to organize my time with Chuck with that in mind.

It's not always smooth sailing, though. At times there will be confusion about living arrangements and difficulty when it's time to say goodbye. These things are sometimes unavoidable. But, if there's anything at all that is good about Alzheimer's, it's that everything is forgotten very quickly. There are no memories of unpleasant events – or of pleasant ones. We always start over with a clean slate.

At seven weeks out, Chuck's transition process appeared to be going along about as well as expected. He seemed a little more willing to accept that we no longer live together, but he still didn't understand why. Leaving him after a visit was less traumatic than it had been a few weeks back, but he wasn't yet comfortable with it. And I couldn't think of a way to make it any easier for him. He always greeted my visits with relief and joy.

"Oh, I'm so glad to see you!"

But my leave-taking was painful, with pleas for me to stay or to let him come with me. Often a staff member had to divert his attention while I made a hurried retreat, but I came every day. He couldn't grasp the fact that he wouldn't be leaving with me. I tried, again and again, to explain that I could no longer take care of him, and he was in good hands where he was. We took walks around the campus, but "walks," meant walking to a favorite bench and sitting there for long periods of time, talking about what a fine day it was, over and over.

But, in two or three months, I started to see a change in him. I began to hear from the staff, and from friends who had visited there, that he seemed to be taking an active part in the activities planned for the residents. I was amazed to hear, for example, that he enjoyed playing Balloon Volleyball. I just couldn't imagine Chuck having fun tossing a balloon back and forth for an hour. I soon found out for myself they were right. Now I often join the game when I'm there; it's actually sort of fun. A few of my fellow residents told me he had recognized them and had greeted them warmly when they went to visit. I noticed that he didn't seem quite so emotional when I had to leave. He would say,

"I wish you wouldn't go. I need you."

But he appeared to accept that I was going, and either retired to his room for a nap, or joined an activity that was in progress.

We had an unusually challenging spring. The weather was unseasonably cold, rainy and gloomy. But the spring flowers, including many kinds of flowering trees and bushes, exploded with color right on cue. Summer arrived more or less on schedule and it was a welcome change. Now, when the weather permitted an outing, we walked outside. I knew Chuck wasn't getting enough exercise, and he seemed to tire after only a short walk. I tried to encourage him to walk a little more, but he soon complained that he was too tired, and wanted to rest. After a while, I gave up trying to be a fitness coach, and admitted defeat. Sooner or later, during our walks, we found ourselves heading for one of the numerous benches placed around the grounds. We settled in there, sometimes for as much as an hour, for "conversation" and an observation of the surrounding scene. They were enjoyable times, in their way. It was peaceful, and I think we both relaxed. In truth, I wanted to cry, thinking about all the good times we've had together. But what good would crying do? Chuck doesn't remember what we've lost, and that is probably just as well. His reality is here and now.

> We sit here side by side, enjoying the sunshine and the cool breezes, but we talk only of the lovely day and the way the wind is moving the trees. It's better than fighting, but I miss you so much. I want to reach out and gather you into my arms. I want it to be the way it used to be, but I know those days are gone forever.

Each time I go to see Chuck, there is more and more evidence that he might be accepting his new life at Harris. He tells anyone who asks how much he likes living there, and he seems willing to remain there when our visit is over. He still sometimes asks where I'm going, but appears to accept that I have a life somewhere else. There are still difficult moments when he gets confused about our living situation. He asks why I don't live with him. I don't feel at all comfortable when I try to explain the reason.

He has connected with the small community at Harris, as well as the staff. He's quick to offer help if someone is having trouble, and he's not shy about expressing his thoughts on some occasions. At lunch one day, we were seated at a table with some residents who appeared quite glum. There were many frowns and grumbles about nothing in particular. After a few minutes, Chuck declared, in a loud voice,

"I have an announcement to make. Everyone at this table has to smile!"

He didn't accomplish his goal, but there were a few startled reactions around the table. I was extremely proud of him. Friends who encounter him during the day, say he is gracious, smiling and seems happy to see them. The staff tells me, "He is a sweet man." He has told more than one visitor,

"There's a charge for visiting here," one of his favorite jokes. One friend told me he now owes Chuck $50.00. I treasure these stories, because they tell me that someday he may no longer be at war with himself or with me. He will have found a place where he feels comfortable. A place where others don't judge him, and where skilled people are able to anticipate his needs and allay his fears. Will he have found more peace than he's had in the last few years? That's a lot to ask, but I will watch and hope for that.

One afternoon, I arrived after lunch and was told he was in his room taking a nap. I knocked and entered his room, where he was stretched out in his chair, customary eye mask in place, and covered by his woolen throw.

"Hi, I came to take you for a walk if you'd like to go. It's a really beautiful day out there."

"Well, sure," he said. "I'd like that."

He rose from his chair, understandably groggy from being asleep, and then said,

"Would it be okay if I just went back to sleep for a little while?" Determined to get him outside, I said,

"Well, why don't we just go outside and sit in the garden and get a little sun? You can always take a nap later."

He seemed to like the idea, so we sat in the garden for about fifteen minutes. When I asked him if he'd like to walk around the campus for a while, he agreed. But as we headed out, he stopped and said,

"I was taking a nap when you came. Would it be all right if I just went back and continued with my nap?"

Of course I agreed, and after I had settled him back in his chair, I kissed him goodbye and left.

After that, I stopped visiting him every day, curious to see if he noticed my absence. With mixed feelings, I observed that, although he was always happy to see me when I arrived, he never seemed aware that I hadn't been there more often. Those who have been through this before, say the experience is typical. It's generally an indication that the transition is working. Chuck may be close to reaching the point where he finally trusts that his caregiving needs will be fulfilled by someone other that me.

Still, back in the corner of my mind where I sometimes push things I'd rather not examine too carefully, there are questions I haven't been asking myself.

> Am I thinking this way because I want so badly for it to be true? Is it really possible that Chuck's transition has been accomplished so quickly and easily? Or am I seeing improvement because I want to see it? I suspect this is going to be much more complicated than it appears now.

Today I think I understand what was causing a large part of his restiveness, angry outbreaks and frequent naps before he moved to Harris. I believe he was scared - scared and insecure. All these things were happening to him and he couldn't understand why. What better way to block it out than to just get into his reclining chair and sleep? It's also quite likely that he was supremely bored. I just wasn't very good at finding things to occupy his attention. Some of the things I thought he might enjoy didn't work out that way at all. Shortly after we moved to Wellman, I learned about a men's discussion group that met on a regular basis. I knew how much Chuck liked good, spirited discussions, so I suggested he try it. After much indecision, he agreed to go, and set off at the appointed time. Fifteen minutes later he was back. When I expressed surprise at his early return, he said,

"All they did was talk about things that weren't very important. Nobody said anything about the world's problems, politics or the economy. I just didn't think it was very interesting."

He used to be a demon Backgammon player (beatable only by his daughter). Now he had no interest in playing at all. I thought if I read to him it might help his comprehension of the news. It worked well for a while, but he couldn't sustain his interest for long, so we stopped. Bridge certainly wasn't a good choice for someone with no memory, so that was out. Occasionally we went to a movie in town; he had no trouble hearing it and it held his attention. But, later on, when I asked if he'd like to see a movie, he answered,

"No, I don't think I want to go. You go."

What he always wanted to do was go out to lunch. So we did at least once, sometimes twice, a week. It always started out well, but soon he would turn to me, with a pained expression, saying,

"What is that noise I hear? It's too noisy in here and it hurts my ears."

Although it was usually nothing much but people at adjoining tables carrying on conversations, or background music – maybe an occasional crash from the kitchen – Chuck solved the problem by removing his hearing aid. That helped cut down on the noise, but it also meant we could no longer carry on a conversation. Soon he began to have difficulty deciding what to order, saying,

"I don't know what I want. You choose."

His ability to handle his utensils and glassware was still quite good, but his food combinations were becoming more imaginative. I watched, fascinated, as he created some of the most unlikely mixtures on his plate and ate them with pleasure.

Eventually, however, his behavior in restaurants gradually changed. He became impatient with the waitress when the food wasn't delivered quickly, or the wine didn't arrive instantly. Soon he forgot that we'd ordered at all, and became annoyed because I wasn't summoning the waiter. All this was easy enough to straighten out, but he often became angry with me when I tried to salvage the situation by explaining that everything was fine.

In the last few years, Chuck has become fascinated by tattoos. I'd never noticed before how many young people who wait on tables have tattoos, but I do now. During one lunch at a local restaurant, he regarded the young woman who was taking our order with great interest.

"What have you got there on your arm?" he said, with eager curiosity.

She murmured something about the tattoo as he continued to gaze at her arm. Then, to my horror, he reached up and gently lifted her sleeve further up her arm.

"Oh, look. It keeps going!"

"Chuck!" I said urgently, "Don't do that. You're embarrassing her!"

He brought his hand away, but gave me a dirty look as he did so. Fortunately, the waitress handled it gracefully, and I was thankful the tattoo had not been on her thigh. And, of course, I was the only one who was embarrassed.

One day I received an email from our credit card bank advising me that a lunch check Chuck had signed included a tip of $20.00, which was exceptionally generous for the cost of the meal we had eaten. He'd always been the one who took care of the bill when we went to restaurants, and I wanted so much for him to feel useful. But I recognized, with great sadness, that still another skill was leaving him. He didn't object when I began picking up the check, but he still makes a point of putting his wallet in his pocket whenever we leave Harris for any reason. His wallet no longer contains a credit card, or much of anything else, but he still wants to make sure that we are prepared to pay the bill. I've noticed that some of the other Harris residents sometimes share that same concern, and worry that they have no money with them to "tip the staff" in the dining room. No amount of assurance that tips are not required and the bill "has been taken care of" seems to convince them, but changing the subject usually solves that problem. I wonder which part of the brain carries that determination to award a provider for services rendered, and why it remains behind after so much else has gone.

TEN

WHERE DO I FIT IN?

I'm still having difficulty figuring out just what my role is, now that I'm no longer Chuck's only caregiver. I know my visits are important to him, and I'm happy to make them. But, when we have lunch at Harris, he reverts to his previous behavior and asks me to order for him. He also wants me to ask the staff for the things he wants. I'm sure he manages when I'm not there, but is he doing this because I am there? The answer to that question is probably, yes, and my presence contributes to it because that was my role at home. There are times when the residents are participating in something they enjoy, such as the monthly art programs we have in conjunction with the local art museum. The staff tries several times to coax him into joining the small group going to the museum, but he won't go unless I explain that I will be there, too. I don't want him to be dependent on me, but I don't want him to think I've abandoned him, either.

As time passes, and I have more opportunities to observe Chuck objectively, I understand more of what's driving some of his behavior patterns. I've read that avoiding shaving, baths and showers is a common characteristic of Alzheimer's. And, sure enough, the staff has been having difficulty convincing him that he needs to take a shower. He simply waves them off, saying,

"I'll do it later."

Recently, a friend asked me,

"Why do people with dementia seem to stop caring about the way they look (and smell, I expect she meant, but didn't say)? They don't seem to care about what clothes they put on or if their hair is combed or not. A lot of them used to be quite fastidious, but now they don't seem to care what they look like."

One has to wonder why those who have always been reasonably well turned out, sometimes turn into individuals who appear to be totally indifferent to personal hygiene. Do they fear some aspect of the shower process, or have they forgotten how to do it? Maybe they view it as an unwelcome break in their routine, or maybe they just don't remember why it's important. Occasionally, when I'm visiting Chuck, I'm able to persuade him to take a shower by gently ordering him to do it. One day, when I suggested that he shower, he said,

"But there isn't a shower in my bathroom."

I reminded him that there were showers, and they were located right next door to his room. He looked surprised, but he accepted it. After he remarked on the lack of shower facilities again one day, I had an idea. I wondered if he believes there are no showers because he doesn't see them. He doesn't have one in his bathroom, where he had always showered in the past, and he doesn't remember where he has been taking a shower at Harris. It's just not a part of his routine yet.

Lately, I've learned that the staff has been trying to coax him into the special whirlpool bath, thinking he will enjoy the experience and, thus, be more agreeable about bathing. At first, he liked it, and stayed there for a luxurious soak. Soon, though, he began to worry that the water was going to overflow the tub and spill out onto the floor. Finally, he resisted going there at all. Today I saw the bathtub for the first time and discovered that it is big, shiny, and bristling with nozzles and nobs of all sorts. I wonder if he's suspicious and a little frightened of the tub. It's entirely possible that, by saying he'll do it later, he's trying to avoid it altogether.

Probably the best answers to my friend's questions about the seeming lack of interest in personal appearance are simple ones. If there were pants and a shirt on the chair next to your bed, why wouldn't you put them on in the morning? You don't remember that you've worn them three days in a row. Your hands may be black with newsprint after you've been reading the paper, but you don't remember why you should go and wash them. When you catch a glimpse of yourself in the bathroom mirror, and you don't recognize who that old person with the messy hair is, why would you pick up a brush and tidy your hair?

The staff is so patient with Chuck, much more so than I would be. They put up with a lot of truculent behavior from some of the residents, without visible consternation. They're able to handle difficult situations with an amazing amount of equanimity. I know this must be difficult to maintain on a regular basis, and I'm sure there is a fair amount of stress that goes with it. But I'm most impressed by their ability to recognize that each resident of Harris is an individual, with individual likes, dislikes and fears. Each person, no matter what degree of dementia has affected his or her brain, is still entitled to respect and dignity. How very fortunate we are that this place exists.

In September, Chuck's sister, Beth, came for a short visit. She lives on the west coast, and it's difficult for her to get away, so we only see her once a year. I was anxious to see if she noticed a difference since she had seen him last.

That had been almost a year ago, when the entire family attended the wedding of his oldest son in Boston. The event had clearly been too much for him. He'd become argumentative, stressed and confused. Beth was immediately struck by how much better he seemed now, and how relaxed he was. She was greatly impressed by the ambiance at Harris, and marveled at how comfortable it looked. He still tended to confuse Beth with his daughter, but he has been doing that for quite a while now. He doesn't see either of them very often, and there is a marked resemblance. We had a pleasant time with Chuck, and the next day we took him out to a local restaurant for lunch. I was interested to note that he didn't bolt his food down as he'd been doing for the past year. In fact, when we have lunch together at Harris, he seems to be eating smaller amounts. He had put on a great deal of weight in the last five or six months, to the point where it had been necessary to buy him new trousers in a larger size. Unfortunately, he has become addicted to vanilla ice cream with chocolate sauce, and it's the high point of his meal. When lunch was over, we drove back to Harris, and Chuck went to take a nap. So far, events had gone smoothly, and Beth was elated to find everything was working so well.

Before she left the next morning, she wanted to say goodbye to Chuck. It was the hour before lunch, when the residents typically begin gravitating toward the dining area. We explained to him several times that we needed to leave shortly because she had to catch a bus, but he was unable to grasp what was happening. He wanted to know where she was going and why. He asked where I was going and when I'd be back. He didn't understand that he was going to have lunch soon, but we wouldn't be joining him. Totally frustrated, he declared,

"I just won't eat lunch, then."

Finally, he insisted on walking with us to the door. At this point, a staff member moved in and gently began talking him toward the dining area. I took my cue, and started to leave, but I could see that Beth was uncertain about what to do and was hanging back, trying to reason with her brother. I motioned for her to join me, which she did, but she was holding back tears as well as she could. As we left, she said,

"I know he's in a good place, but I feel so sorry for him."

I understood what she was feeling, but I said,

"Please don't be sorry; he's going to be fine. In a few minutes he will have forgotten everything that happened."

When I saw him the next day, he didn't remember that Beth had been here.

At lunchtime today, Chuck was a bit crabby at times; he appeared a little more confused than normal, and frequently employed a gesture that's been characteristic of him for the last few years. It means, basically,

"Surely you don't expect me to accept that!"

Fortunately, the weather today was a typical, perfect fall day, with sun, blue skies and a cool, stiff breeze. It was a welcome change from the hot, muggy days we'd suffered through all week. We took a walk up to our favorite spot at the highest point on campus, and sat contentedly in the sun. I asked him, as casually as I could,

"Would you like it better if I didn't come and have lunch with you?"

He looked at me with concern, and said,

"Oh, no. I love it when you come!"

I mentioned that he seemed a little cross and I wondered if he would rather I hadn't come today.

"I'm not cross at all," he said, "I love seeing you."

I decided to leave it there. As he began to relax and enjoy the spectacular day we were having, he gradually became more like the old Chuck, laughing and teasing. We stayed for quite a while, talking a lot about the wind and the falling leaves, but settling in to a feeling of shared contentment. I realized it had been a long time since I had genuinely enjoyed being with him. There was no tension, no anger and no insecurity, and we were free to enjoy each other again. Although I know there will still be times ahead when it will be quite different, I'm grateful for these occasional bright spots, and I marvel that they are still there.

Erica told me today that people with Alzheimer's are often more likely to lash out at the ones they love. That would certainly explain the annoyed looks and the scolding I often get when we're with others. I suppose Chuck feels more comfortable taking out his frustrations on me because I'm the one he knows the best. Maybe I provide an outlet for the insecurities and confusion he feels at times.

> Why do you get so annoyed with me? You seemed ashamed of me when we're around other people, and I don't understand why. It would be easy to explain it by assuming you are angry with me because you blame me for bringing you here. But I think that's just me feeling guilty; I believe it's something you don't understand and you have lost the ability to tell me what it is.

When the time came for his customary nap, we returned to his room, where he settled into his chair. As I bent over to give him a kiss, he grabbed my shoulders and said,

"Will you marry me?" I kissed him and said, "I thought you'd never ask."

ELEVEN

THE CAREGIVER'S DILEMMA

Could Chuck's transition really be happening this quickly? I'd hoped it would successfully take place, and I had fervently wanted it to. Now that it seems likely, I'm flooded with all sorts of emotions. For several years, I've taken on the role of his caregiver. Suddenly, my job appears to have changed radically. I'm having a hard time figuring out how to think about that, but the truth is, my caregiver job is over.

Or is it? When I began visiting Chuck after the transition, I had tried to be as upbeat as I could. I guess I was hoping he would somehow understand that our situation was better now, and I could go back to being his wife again. After several days, however, I'd stopped telling myself our relationship would improve much. I'd lost sight of the fact that he'd forgotten there was anything wrong with it.

I wonder if I'll ever completely come to terms with the reality of this disease. You can learn everything there is to know about Alzheimer's. You can talk with people who've gone through it, and listen to professionals who have devoted their careers to caring for those who have it. But it's extremely difficult to apply all that knowledge to yourself and your husband. Does anyone ever really learn to accept the hard facts? This disease will steadily get worse, and it's terminal. I know these things, but I'm still having trouble convincing myself. I've reached the point where I can accept that the transition is working, but I'm also beginning to realize just how much of my life in the last few years has been defined by being a caregiver. I am so thankful that this place exists, and that we're able to reap the benefits, but it's hard for me to figure out where I belong at this stage of the journey.

Directly after the transition started, I still reeled with the effects of the upheaval, but I felt as if I had finally let out a tremendous breath of air - one I'd been holding in for a long time. I'd gone through a sort of trial by fire and come out on the other side. The people who were caring for Chuck really understood what he needed and how to meet those needs. I was finally free to spend my time any way I wanted to. I spent a lot of it re-arranging the furniture in the apartment to reflect its new single-occupancy status; being fully aware that I was also trying to re-arrange the past as soon as I could. I bought season tickets to lectures and concerts, and joined friends for lunch or dinner. I even took a quick trip into New York City. The feeling was disconcertingly similar to the time after my divorce many years ago. I had moved into my own apartment in Greenwich Village, excited by my new life. This time, though, it's not the same. This time I fear I've lost more than I've gained, but I also feel liberated.

It takes a while to realize that the Alzheimer's journey isn't over just because your husband has reached the safety of the dementia care facility. You don't simply hand him over to others and say,

"Okay, now he's your problem."

Now I need to learn how I can engage with him without being too intrusive. I try to make frequent visits; some go quite well, others not so well. It appears his new routine is well on the way to becoming acceptable. He is always happy to see me, and we usually spend the time sitting and talking either in a quiet spot, in his room or outside when the weather is good. I try to talk about things I think will interest him, whether it's a lecture I've attended or something I've read. He listens carefully for a while, but it's obvious he's not processing much of what I'm telling him. I'm not surprised when he loses interest and shifts to another thought.

I talked to Dr. Gordon today, and told her about the "conversations" I try to have with Chuck. He seems unable to talk about anything but the weather. Although he does answer the questions I ask him, he doesn't take it any farther than that. Also, I'm not sure how important my visits are to him now. She explained that he has reached the stage where his brain is losing the capacity to initiate topics for discussion and, from now on, I will need to fill that role. As for the importance of my visits, she suggested I talk to the staff and learn what they've observed. Shortly after she called, I received an email from her, saying she had called Erica about my question, and was told my visits are very important to Chuck. Erica wondered if I could share a meal with him more often; mealtime is often when he asks where I am.

Dr. Gordon also told me she had recently asked a physician in residence at the hospital to meet Chuck and talk with him for a while. Said physician happened to be an attractive young woman who had never been to Harris before. After they were introduced, Chuck assumed the role of gracious host. He took her on a tour of the facility, showed her his room, and was most animated and talkative. When she asked him if this was a good place to live, he assured her that it was a wonderful place and he enjoyed living there. I was amazed when I heard that, but then I remembered that this was one of the skills at which he used to excel. I expect he really meant it at the time, and I chuckled when I imagined the conversation.

At first, I tried to look for places where we could talk quietly in private when I went to visit him. Soon I realized that he welcomes the appearance of others, and tries his best to get them to join us. He seems to enjoy talking to people, hearing about them and telling them things about himself. He asks them the same questions more than once, in spite of having just heard the answers. Mostly, they take that in stride, and tell him again.

What is happening here? Why does he prefer to include others in our discussions when our time together is so important? Maybe it isn't as important to him as it is to me. I think about it a lot, but can only come up with conjectures. Is it because he doesn't know how to think about our relationship now, and feels more comfortable with others around? Or is it possible that he is dimly aware that he's not able to carry on conversations with me and needs someone else to help out? Could it be that he's now so accustomed to being with other people all the time that he feels uncomfortable when he's alone with me? Or is this simply the way he is today, and I should spend less time worrying about it?

A few days ago, I read a newspaper article about a group of neuroscientists who are studying the way human brains perceive and react to stimulus. One part that caught my attention explained that social connections are important to us because we learn by imitating the behavior of others. We feel more comfortable experiencing events with a group than we do when we are alone. I wonder if Chuck has been living with the Harris residents long enough so that he feels more comfortable and secure with them than he does when he's alone with me. It makes a lot of sense, particularly for someone with Alzheimer's who's insecure about his place in the world and is having trouble understanding what is happening to him.

Recently, I've noticed that Chuck's impatience with me has increased, especially when we're around other people. I'm not sure what's driving this behavior; maybe this is his attempt to understand where I belong in his new life. Often, when I'm at Harris for lunch, I notice that he becomes rather critical of some of the residents' behavior, and his attempts to call it to their attention are, shall we say, somewhat misguided. But if I try to intercede in any of these situations, I'm treated to a lot of frowning and eye rolling.

But he does seem happier now; I can see it when I'm able to observe him before he's aware I have arrived. He has others to talk and joke with. His every need and want is taken care of. He still has his beloved glass of bourbon (at somewhat less than full strength) every evening, which is served to him by the nurse who distributes the medications. It had to be prescribed for him! We had a big lunchtime party to celebrate his 86th birthday, complete with balloons, singing, presents and a giant chocolate cake with chocolate icing and his name spelled out on top. He reveled in the attention and the fuss being made over him and, when it was all over, he went off to take a nap. As I tucked him in, he said,

"I love you, and I need you." I replied as lightly as I could,

"No, you don't need me so much any more, but I hope you never stop loving me."

He just smiled and said, "I'll always love you."

I know there are people who, once they have placed their spouse in a dementia care facility, have never quite been able to shake off the feeling that they've done him a terrible wrong. They are convinced he hates it there and wants only to go home. Perhaps they've forgotten how painful their lives were before they made the transition. Maybe they haven't allowed themselves to think about the adjustment that he will inevitably make. I think part of it may be guilt about feeling relief from the burden of caregiving.

"I'm his wife. I'm supposed to look after him!" There may also be a slight feeling of rejection.

"I changed my whole way of life for him; now he acts like he doesn't need me any more."

Maybe they're beginning to realize that their role isn't going to be the same any more. They've been so caught up with caregiving that they haven't had a chance to think about what happens next.

I've thoroughly enjoyed the freedom to do what I want, but curiously, for a while after Chuck left, I felt as if I'd lost my anchor and was aimlessly drifting. I suppose this drifting sensation was a natural reaction to the sudden change in my position as caregiver – similar to the one you have when you've just been fired. I think, too, that it reflects something more urgent. Now that I have all this free time, what will I do with it?

If we have spent most of the last few years being a caregiver, it may gradually occur to us that we now have a void to fill. We'll have to find something to give additional purpose to our lives. We may be too old to get a job, but we're never too old to continue our education. Think of the possibilities! We now have the time to go back to school (Oldest Graduate in the U.S.!), take up painting, learn to make pots on a wheel, write our memoirs, travel to places we've never seen. Or, if that's too ambitious, sing in a choir, read all those books we never had time for, or volunteer some of our newfound time to a cause we believe in. Now we can go to all those movies and concerts that our husbands would have hated.

I've gradually become reconciled to the fact that I'm losing to Alzheimer's the man with whom I've now shared most of my life. I've spent some tearful moments remembering our marriage as a connection between two people who love each other deeply. We each knew we'd filled a great need in the other. We'd believed this to be a bond between us capable of withstanding almost anything. But is that bond still there? Now that I'm no longer his caregiver, I am free to be his wife. But what does that mean? I seem to be living in two worlds now. There's my life on the outside, where I go about my business as if everything were the same. And there's the life where I visit a husband whom I love and I miss – a husband who is drifting farther and farther away, and now has a separate existence that doesn't really include me any more.

As children, we were told you couldn't eat your cake and have it, too. We were too young then to grasp the message implied there, that we would someday need to make hard decisions with ramifications that might be very uncomfortable. We only learn those truths much later in life. My truth may simply be that I've made a tradeoff. I've traded spending the rest of our lives together for Chuck's feeling of security and my tranquility. For a while, I had forgotten how much I love him. I rejoice in the return of that love, but it has come at a high price.

> Wait a minute! There seems to be an overabundance of self-pity going on here! Every time I begin to think this way, I need to stop and think about what our lives would be like now if Chuck hadn't gone to Harris. I need to remember all those mornings when I lay in bed, dreading the day ahead; and the afternoons that almost always went from bad to worse. We were gradually becoming characters in a Greek tragedy; deprived of the ability to enjoy the time we have left.

Some days go better than others. I've worked out the best times to visit Chuck, and I try to stick with that schedule as much as I can. I join him for lunch at Harris three times a week, and I try to get there at least one other day. Are they pleasant occasions? Not particularly, but I think he likes having me come. It's during these times that I feel the most confused about what I'm supposed to be doing.

We often share a table with other residents who are in varying stages of dementia. They recognize me now, although I doubt they entirely understand who I am or what I'm doing there. I feel a great deal of empathy with them, because I think I have some idea of what they're experiencing. I try to engage them in conversation, or at least give them a hug or pat on the back. Sometimes they look at me with such endearing smiles that I wish I knew what they're thinking.

Chuck has developed a heightened concern for the welfare of his fellow residents. As a result, he's sometimes over-solicitous about making sure they get the help they need, often to the point where he just adds to the confusion. Should I chastise him for trying to help? I know he's desperate to find a role for himself in this new environment. I believe the staff understands this, but I feel awkward just sitting there, doing nothing. It makes me feel guilty to have the staff waiting on me at lunchtime, when I know they're busy and I could easily give them a hand. Erica tells me it's possible that I'm using this as an excuse to get away from a strained environment for a little while. These are all situations I've never had to think about before, so I have no precedents to guide me.

But something else has occurred to me recently. I've been spending so much time worrying about my place in Chuck's care process that I've been neglecting to think about it from his point of view. Is it possible that some of his behavior toward me might be reflecting his own doubt about my role? Could it be that I'm not the only one who's doubtful about what I'm supposed to be doing? Maybe he's confused about it, too. Maybe he doesn't know how to think about me anymore.

TWELVE

I NEED YOU

Chuck has been at Harris for a year now. He seems to have adjusted to life there remarkably well. But the time when I need to leave is still the most difficult part of the visit. Always, following lunch, he is ready to take a nap. After we go through the ritual of getting him settled in his reclining chair, I give him a kiss and leave without further ado. But sometimes he becomes more insistent, asking me,

"When will I see you next?"

I try to come up with an answer that satisfies him, but it doesn't always work. With urgency in his voice, he says,

"Just tell me what your plans are. I need to know the plan." That seems to be a major worry right now, and I'm guessing that it's one of the things that concern many with dementia. At Harris there is a large message board, prominently displayed, that lists all of the day's activities and what time they will happen. The things on the list may not be fully understood by the residents, and they may not be interested in attending them all, but they represent signposts that help organize the time into manageable bits.

Yesterday, Chuck seemed unusually agitated, and he begged me to take him "home".

"I don't understand why I have to be here. I need you."

This has happened more than once and, if I'm not careful, the conversation will continue as follows:

"I just want to go home with you. I need you, and I don't belong here; I want to go back home."

Although he sometimes says he wants to leave, he has never said that he doesn't like Harris, or that he is unhappy here. I don't believe he has any concept of where "here" is; I don't think any of the residents do. It's simply the world in which they exist. These conversations bothered me a lot in the beginning, because they tapped into the fathomless well of guilt that is always there below the surface. But gradually I began to understand that, when Chuck says he wants to go home, what he really means is that he wants to return to the way he was before Alzheimer's took over his life. Possibly, he's able to recall some distant memory of how he was in the past, enough to know that it was better then than it is now. It's futile to explain to him that we can never return to "the way it was before". Our lives have changed. He's here because the care he needs is beyond what I can give him now, and it's this way for keeps. It will always be necessary for me to tell him that, and he will never understand.

After one particularly uncomfortable attempt to say goodbye to Chuck, shortly before dinnertime one evening, he somehow managed to follow me through the main door before the automatic lock clicked on. He followed me down the hall, shouting that he was coming with me, and nothing I said could persuade him otherwise. Two of the staff members had followed him. We were all trying to figure out how to calm him down and get him to turn around and come back. We were failing dismally; he was becoming more and more distraught. Just then a friend came into view. He sized up the situation, threw his arm around Chuck, and said,

"Hey, Chuck, let's go get some dinner!"

With that, they walked off, Chuck in great spirits, forgetting all that had just happened. It was obvious to me that, from then on, I would need to schedule my visits so I can leave at a time when he is otherwise occupied. These episodes, although disquieting, are part of my learning experience. I'm still feeling my way, but

I wonder if I will ever reach the point where I can handle things with equanimity.

This afternoon I had a call from Julie, the nurse at Harris. She told me that Chuck was unusually agitated and seemed to be convinced that something terrible had happened to me. I said I'd be right down. When I arrived, he was still agitated, and he was angry. I tried to find out why he was so upset with me, but he was unable to tell me. Finally, I managed to persuade him to go back to his room with me and talk about it. As near as I could determine, he was angry because he thought I'd abruptly walked out on him without telling him when I would return. He said,
 "I would never do that to you."
 I tried to tell him that I'd spent some time with him the previous day, and had told him many times when I would be coming again. I knew it was useless to remind him; he wasn't capable of remembering. But I sensed he thought we were having an intelligent conversation, and were talking out a problem the way we had always done in the past. By the time I left, he seemed to have regained his composure. We said goodbye, and he went to join the group of residents who were having afternoon tea and cookies.
 What caused that outburst? Apparently he had been quietly reading the newspaper when he

suddenly got up and started shouting that he knew something terrible had happened to me. He became agitated when he couldn't make the staff understand. We will never know what triggered that horrifying conviction. What was happening inside that ravaged brain?

But that episode gave me an idea for something that might help. I used to leave him notes on the hall mirror in our apartment, telling him where I was going and when I'd be back. It might work again. I bought a small whiteboard, the kind you can wipe off each time you want to write something new. We mounted it on the door to his bathroom where he would always see it. Now, each time I leave him after a visit, I write what day and time I'll be back again. So far, it has worked quite well. There aren't as many phone calls from him, asking when I'm coming. He knows it's written on the board, and he (and the staff) can get his answer there. But I don't know how long it will be effective.

Another interesting situation has developed recently. For some reason I can't figure out, he sometimes believes he's on a boat, and he thinks I am, too. When he doesn't see me, he fears something bad has happened, and he desperately needs to find me. When he can't make anyone understand what he wants, he becomes quite agitated – sometimes angry. The first time it happened, a staff member panicked and telephoned me. I spoke with Chuck, but he was too upset to understand what I was saying. What is worse, I don't think he was wearing his hearing aid. Fortunately, Erica picked up the phone and assured me that she would work with him until he felt comfortable.

Eventually, the staff became familiar with these episodes, and helped him to work his way through them. Chuck spent four years in the Navy, we owned a small boat at one time, and we have taken many small boat cruises in the course of our travels. Could that be the basis for these boat fantasies? Oddly, I've heard of several instances when an individual suffering from dementia has imagined himself on a boat at sea. I wonder if it's just coincidental, or if there might be a common denominator there.

When Chuck says, "I need you" he means it, but it's nothing new. He has always needed me, and I him. We've each had many good friends in our lives, but after we married, we became each other's best friend. I learned to understand how much he depended on me for the emotional security that he had apparently never had. In return, he believed in me and gave me the self-confidence to believe in myself. Those were our gifts to each other. And so, instead of trying to explain all of that to him, I kiss him goodbye and tell him I love him and I will never be very far from him. I firmly believe that, no matter how difficult things become, it will always be important that he knows how much I love him.

Taking advantage of my newfound freedom, I traveled last winter to Tanzania. Chuck and I have been to Africa three times, because we could never get enough of it. I went back with mixed feelings about going this time. I travelled with his daughter, but it seemed strange to go there without Chuck. I missed sharing the adventure with him, and imagined the joy he would have felt. But as I went through the familiar experience of looking for the animals, meeting the Tanzanian people and learning about their lives, I was finally able to start thinking realistically about our situation. Yes, Chuck would have loved seeing lions, elephants and zebra again, and the beautiful, mystical landscape of Africa. But he has lost the ability to put up with the uncomfortable aspects of the trip: the long plane rides, the bumpy and dusty roads, the occasionally primitive plumbing and the need to stay on schedule.

He would no longer enjoy the jockeying for position it takes to get the perfect photo of a rhinoceros, or have the patience to look for common interests among the crazy quilt of personalities that made up our tour group. Things he was once happy to endure for the sake of the experience would now infuriate him and would be beyond his ability to understand.

Above all, he needs the security of knowing what is coming next. Routine is his lifeline now. Finally, he would have had no memories to cherish of a wonderful adventure. I see that now, and it's helping me to think in a way that is more realistic.

I lay awake one night during that trip, listening to the sounds of Africa. I heard the rumble of a nearby lioness, reminding us that she was here, too. There was no mistaking the dissonant serenade of the hyenas – always there, waiting. It was then that I remembered what it was about hyenas I don't like. Unlike most African predators, who kill their prey before devouring it, hyenas leap onto their victim while it's running away. They begin eating the animal while it's still alive. It's hard to resist the comparison with Alzheimer's.

It's time to stop dwelling on the fact that the man I fell in love with so many years ago has all but disappeared. Deep below the surface of that confused and often unhappy person we see now, is the Chuck I still remember so well. That's the man I want to remember. I try not to lose sight of that. I knew my husband very well. I understood him well enough to know that radical change was not something he embraced easily. He made life-changing decisions only when he felt strongly that they were right. He was strong, reliable, trustworthy, and had infinite faith in his convictions. How much of that man remains today?

That's how Alzheimer's works. It's the hyena, gradually eating away the brain cells, removing memory forever. It also destroys the parts of the brain where judgment, confidence and courage reside, leaving only a slough of uncertainty. Chuck is sinking into that slough, but I know he will not go easily. Each time he struggles to keep from going under, I will understand what's happening. He will not give up without a fight.

THIRTEEN

HOW TO AVOID LEARNING THE HARD WAY

If you are just beginning to care for someone with dementia, you can be easily overwhelmed by the scope of the job. At this point in the narrative, I'd like to share some of the things I've learned while I've been a caregiver. You may find them helpful.

    Two or three years before we moved to Wellman, I had already recognized one way I could make life easier for both of us – I could assume responsibility for the household finances. Paying bills, balancing the checkbook, keeping track of various payments, that kind of thing. Chuck was happy to have me do it, and turned the job over with relief. Each family has their own method of dealing with these tasks, but there are some areas that you should begin to explore before much more time passes. Maybe you are already the one who pays the bills and looks after financial details in your household, in which case you can skim through the next part. If your spouse has always handled this job in the past, read on.

Today's women are at a definite advantage over their mother and grandmother's generation. Thankfully, we're past the days when it was assumed that women didn't need to "bother their pretty little heads" with financial matters. Traditionally, this job had always been the responsibility of the Man of the House, at least in my generation. But some time ago we all began to recognize that a woman could handle the job every bit as well as a man, and sometimes better. Today, many of us are quite comfortable with ruling the financial realms of a household.

As you start to see signs that your husband is becoming less capable of dealing with these tasks, you should begin to educate yourself about the intricacies of these responsibilities. Do you both have up-to-date wills, do you know where they are, and have you read them? Will you have General Power of Attorney when it becomes necessary? Do you have Advanced Directives for Health Care? If you do, are you the one responsible for your husband's health care decisions if he can no longer make them himself? If he is responsible for decisions about your health care when you can't make them anymore, it's time to change that.

If there's an investment account, who manages it and in whose name is the account?

Are you familiar with your bank accounts and credit card accounts? Who generally pays the bills in your household and how are they paid – by mail or online? Who does your tax returns, and where are the forms and supporting documents required to prepare them? Are there family trusts or other funds you should know more about?

    I'm not trying to scare you, but these are things you should know, and now is a good time to start learning about them. If your husband is capable of filling you in on what needs to be done, wonderful; but this discussion assumes that capability may no longer be in play. You might begin by sitting down with your lawyer and asking questions. If there are investment accounts, you'll need to schedule an appointment with the accounts manager, who should be happy to make sure you understand how the accounts have been set up, and the role you'll need to play in the future. If you are terrified by all of the above, you can seek out a family member or an old, trusted friend and tell her or him your concerns. If you have confidence in that person, it will be a great relief to have someone who gives you moral support and can help you find your way. If none of the above works for you, you can turn it all over to someone who is skilled at handling these responsibilities – for a fee.

For many people with Alzheimer's, one of the more distressing manifestations can be paranoia. In that case, your husband is likely to become suspicious and agitated by any interest you are suddenly showing in matters that have always been his domain. If this happens to you, you'll have to carry out your research in a way that doesn't excite suspicion. I'm not advocating creeping around behind the furniture. That makes you feel guilty and sneaky, and you have enough on your mind as it is. You'll figure out how to learn what you need to know in the way that works best for you.

There is an eventual happy ending to all of this. Once you have started taking over some of the more challenging household responsibilities, you may find your husband is actually grateful. He may have been aware that he could no longer fill that role and, once he feels you can handle it, he might relax and stop worrying. Better still, you may find you actually enjoy doing these things. Now that you've found out how everything works, you can have more confidence in yourself and enjoy the empowerment that goes along with it. When that day comes, you can congratulate yourself on reaching a meaningful milestone.

Above all, you should begin to think about yourself. You're going to hear that a lot, but it's true. Are you spending all of your time being a caregiver? If it hasn't happened already, you will undoubtedly suffer from constant exposure to what is, at best, a difficult situation. Many women have been conditioned by tradition to think they must be the sole caregivers for a loved one. Most of us have been partners for a long time in marriages that were based on love and trust. The idea of turning your husband over to someone you'll pay to take care of him, is more than distasteful, it's unthinkable. But imagine yourself in any of the following situations.

You've stopped going out to lunch with friends. You don't go to movies or concerts anymore. You haven't gone to your book club discussions in months. You missed your last school reunion, and you've lost touch with most of your classmates. You don't see much of your children these days, and your grandchildren are growing up too fast for you to keep track of.

You've started to have headaches that sometimes linger for more than a day or two, and you're told it's probably because you clench your teeth when you sleep. You have always been a sound sleeper, but now you wake up in the middle of the night and can't get back to sleep. How about that cold you had, that steadily got worse until you were afraid it might be flu or pneumonia? You fell and sprained your ankle, and it's taking a long time to heal. You seem to burst into tears for no reason at all. You haven't seen a doctor because you can't take the time off.

Please keep this in mind. If you continue along your present path with no relief, you will almost certainly turn into a person you do not like. There's a good chance you will become so stressed that you'll need medical care, and maybe even end up in the hospital. As a result, you won't be a help to anybody. You'll make a bad situation even worse. You Must Have Help!

It's quite likely that your children will not be a part of the solution. Either they live too far away or they have full time jobs. They are raising families, and their children take up most of their spare time. For several reasons that may not surprise you, it's quite likely that they really don't want to take on a caregiver job. But you most certainly should have this discussion with your family. It's extremely important that they be aware of the enormity of the job you are facing.

Fortunately, you have other options open to you for getting help. There are several resources you can tap for good, trustworthy part-time caregivers. Ask around for the names of people with good references. Try your doctor, the telephone directory, the Internet, people you know who have employed caregivers. Then interview them and try it out. You may have luck with the first one you hire; if not, keep trying. Having someone who can take over for a while is a precious asset. At the least, you'll gain an hour or two for yourself, out of the house, doing something you enjoy. At best, your husband might enjoy the company of someone new occasionally. And it will give you time to find a hassle-free vantage point. From there, you can assess your situation and make intelligent decisions about what to do next.

Now that I've just told you what you need to do, I must reveal that Chuck decided, early in the above process, that he wanted no part of a part-time caregiver. I had been referred to Sally, a remarkable woman with whom I found an instant rapport. She was warm, attractive and intelligent, and she was quite familiar with Alzheimer's care. I described her to Chuck, who wanted to know why we needed her.

"She'll be someone for you to talk to, maybe even go for an occasional walk with," I said.

"Well, I don't need anyone to talk to; I have you," he replied.

"Yes," I said, "but wouldn't it be nice if you occasionally had someone besides me to talk to?"

He grudgingly agreed, mostly to please me, I'm sure, and we set up a date with Sally. She stayed with him for an hour, while I went to the library. When I returned, I asked him how it had gone.

"Oh, fine." he said, "She seems like a nice person."

I was understandably overjoyed, and looked forward to making this a weekly, maybe even twice-weekly, event when I could get away occasionally. But it was not to be. Sally had told me Chuck was a delight to talk to and a very nice man; she said he seemed to enjoy their conversations. After her next visit, the following week, I asked Chuck again if he had enjoyed it.

"It was all right," he said, "but I didn't learn anything."

When the time came to schedule another visit, he said he thought it was a waste of time.

"We never get anywhere in our conversations," he said. "I don't see any point in it. I don't need a babysitter."

I explained, somewhat testily, that there wasn't meant to be a "point in it". It was more of an occasional opportunity for companionship with someone else. He, of course, saw no reason for someone else – that was my role. But it does work for many people, and I urge you to try it.

One way to carve out some relief time for yourself might be to find someone who could come in and read aloud from books or periodicals your husband enjoys. Try locating a high-school student who would be willing to play chess or some other board game after school. How about asking an old friend to stop by and reminisce about old times. (It doesn't matter if memories aren't 100% accurate!) Connect with someone who shares a common sports interest and suggest they occasionally attend a sports event together, with the tickets on you. Does your husband enjoy watching television? If so, that opens up quite a few possibilities, assuming he is willing to do it. It might be wise to make sure that he still remembers how to work the remote. Unfortunately, that's often one of the first skills to disappear.

I tried movies on TV I thought Chuck might like – not an easy task – but the problem was hearing and comprehension. I found that closed captions or subtitles helped a great deal. Seeing the words made a lot of difference in his understanding of what was happening on the screen. Unfortunately, not all the movies I wanted came with those features. I had to pass up some movies I knew he would enjoy, mostly because the dialogue was too fast for him, or the actors had foreign accents. If he couldn't figure out what the movie was about, there wasn't much point in sitting through it. And so he didn't.

He did, however, love to watch tennis and football on TV. He always asked if there was a game on, but he was mostly interested in his beloved Patriots. He would stick with a football game the longest of anything on television and, for a while, he watched games even if I didn't watch with him. I'm far from being a devoted football fan, but I didn't mind watching the important games with him. It provided a welcome opportunity to share time without bickering or long, empty silences.

Did he used to play tennis? I've discovered there are televised tennis matches going on somewhere, almost every week of the year. The major tournaments, which begin in March and continue through September, are covered by a tennis channel and are exciting to watch. If you have a recording device with your television set, you can tape the matches and watch them whenever you want – without commercials.

If your husband was once a golfer, I've found that a good tournament on TV might hold his interest for a while. As an added enhancement, the hushed commentary and slow pace will eventually put both of you to sleep. The Masters Tournament, in April, is always fun to watch. The players are good, there are few commercial messages and the golf course is spectacularly beautiful.

Now it might be a good idea to talk about the Cocktail Hour and the "cocktail" part of it. Alcohol is a subject that may be necessary to think about, particularly if it has been a part of your normal routine for a while. I expect you'll know if it applies to your situation. We all know that none of us can, or should, drink the same amount of alcohol we did when we were younger, but what about a person with Alzheimer's? I won't attempt to give you advice on this matter. That is best done by your primary care physician, and depends greatly on the circumstances of each individual. I will, however, tell you what we did.

    We had always enjoyed an evening cocktail or two, as well as wine with dinner. I was advised to reduce the amounts to one glass of each for both of us. Chuck was a bourbon drinker, and he liked it strong, with very little ice. I watched carefully to see if it seemed to affect him much, which was difficult during the period when he was angry a great deal of the time. I couldn't be certain if he was worse when he drank his stiff bourbon, but I decided to see if cutting back might make him a little less contentious. I began by offering to make the cocktails every evening, and he happily agreed. I didn't have much success with adding more water to his drink; he complained right away that it was too weak. Finally, I resorted to something I thought I would never do. Surreptitiously, I started adding water to the bourbon bottle; a little at first, and then progressively more until it was diluted almost by half. It solved the puzzle of how to minimize the alcohol level. Surprisingly, maybe because he saw it being poured from the bottle, he didn't seem to notice it was weaker. We solved the wine situation by using the same technique. I tried serving alcohol-free wine for a while, but we both thought it tasted terrible. Water in the wine worked fine, especially if one of us didn't know the difference. I can't be sure, though, that all this subterfuge had much, if any, effect on his general demeanor.

In the beginning, these deceptions bothered me a great deal. We have always been honest with each other, and it was hard to imagine thinking any other way. But perplexing problems sometimes call for subtle solutions. I learned early on that any harmony in our day-to-day existence depended on avoiding circumstances that led to altercation. I reasoned that, although I wasn't being entirely straightforward in some areas, it was far better than courting certain strife. I believed it was the best way to handle the problem, but I didn't feel any sense of accomplishment. What I felt was more like guilt.

FOURTEEN

A LONG ILLNESS

This week we received news that a college classmate and friend had died, "...after a long illness." We knew he had Alzheimer's, which most probably led to his death. Why didn't the obituary tell us that? If it was the family's decision to omit that information, I support their right to do so, but it makes me wonder. Would knowing this about his death diminish his life in any way? Would it take away all of the many remarkable things he was able to accomplish? Would it make us forget what a good friend and loving husband he was? If we're going to fight this disease, we can't be afraid to acknowledge it. In order to accomplish that goal, we're going to have to call it what it is. At present, Alzheimer's appears to be a terrible side effect of living longer than our ancestors did. It's a problem we must work to solve, because right now, anyone who has the disease, or will have it soon, has no chance to survive it.

Remember when cancer was a forbidden subject? A diagnosis was tantamount to a death sentence, and it was a long time before we were able to discuss "the C word" in anything but hushed and horrified tones. But as more and more people were stricken with it, and successful treatments began to emerge, we started treating cancer like an enemy we had to conquer. We learned more about it, discussed it freely, and now it enjoys more fund raising events and publicity, enabling more research breakthroughs, than any other disease today.

When will we see the same thing happening for Alzheimer's? At present, Alzheimer's is a disease with only minimal treatment available and no cure in sight. No one recovers from it, and it's a leading cause of death in recent years, far outpacing heart disease and cancer. We are told it can be inherited and, if a parent or a grandparent had it, there's a strong possibility that you will get it, too. And, as if that isn't enough bad news: outside of a very few characteristics known about the disease, no one is really sure yet what causes it. Doesn't that sound to you like something we should be fighting to change? Where are the "Races for the Cure", the telethons, the ribbon loops, and efforts to involve the public in this cause?

Today we are faced with still another problem – the outrageous cost of health care in this country. No doubt we will build more continuing care communities for all those growing numbers of seniors, but how many of them can afford to live there? Most of those facilities will probably include care for dementia patients. But will there be enough medical professionals to staff them? We're being told that registered nurses and licensed practical nurses are already in short supply. Are we destined to return to the Old Folks' Homes or the Poor Houses of our past? One thing is certain. There will always be a need for caregivers.

Part of the reason why we avoid talking about Alzheimer's when we begin to age, is because it has started to feel like more of a threat than it did before. It has become something we fear, but which is largely unacknowledged. Unlike cancer, children and young adults don't get Alzheimer's; it only appears when we are old, so it's easy to ignore unless it happens to someone close to us. We live in a society that fears getting old. Some of the reasons that keep us from visiting people with dementia reflect that fear. If you have been thinking some of these things, you are not alone:

"I don't know what to expect from people with dementia, how to talk to them, or even how to think about them. I wouldn't know how to act around them."

"I worry that I will be a candidate for dementia someday, and I'm not ready to think about that yet."

"I don't really understand Alzheimer's, but I know what it does to people and how it turns out. These people remind me of something I'd prefer not to acknowledge right now."

I have no doubt that research will eventually discover more effective treatments and even a prevention for Alzheimer's, but it won't be any time soon. In the meantime, we can help by talking openly about this disease that has changed our loved ones into strangers. An acquaintance, upon hearing from me that my husband has Alzheimer's, remarked with great surprise,

"But isn't there a pill for that?"

We can help to dispel some of the beliefs that others have, by supplying accurate information and gently dispelling the misconceptions.

In the meantime, according to the Alzheimer's Association, more than five million Americans have Alzheimer's and more than fifteen million (mostly unpaid) individuals spend an estimated 18.2 billion hours caring for them. Those numbers will grow much larger soon. The Baby Boomer generation will soon reach 70 and 80, the age at which Alzheimer's is most likely to appear. As a result, our society will soon face a major disaster. Is the medical profession equal to the task? Are our existing caregiving facilities adequate to meet the demand, and will everyone be able to afford them? Who will pay for the research needed to figure out what causes this disease and how we can treat it? Or will Alzheimer's continue to be something we avoid thinking and talking about, hoping we won't get it, while millions of people stand helplessly by, watching their loved ones gradually disappear?

FIFTEEN

ALL THE HELP WE CAN GET

When Chuck began the transition to Harris, I never intended to keep his whereabouts a secret, and I told anyone who asked, where he had gone. Soon, I began to hear from people in the Wellman community who wanted to know if I'd be willing to talk with them about our experience. All of them were people who were caring for a partner with dementia, and nearly all of them were miserable. The questions they asked reflected the urgency of their concerns:

"When did you first know he had Alzheimer's?"

"How did you know when it was time to go to Harris?"

"Now that my husband is in long-term care, what should I be doing?"

"I feel so badly about my wife, but I'm not doing a very good job of taking care of her."

"My life is hell, but I feel guilty for thinking that way because his is worse."

One by one, I shared my experiences with the people who asked, and listened as they told me about theirs. Occasionally, when we met in the halls, I would ask how things were going and we would often talk for several minutes. In time, one of them called me and asked me to join a group of women who were planning to meet for coffee on Saturday morning to discuss caregiver issues. That was the beginning of a small session we have held every Saturday morning since. We trade experiences, share personal stories, shed a few tears and, most important, we provide support for each other – confident that what we say will never leave the room. We never know how many of us are suffering quietly and alone, until they tell us. So, one way or another, we need to find each other and, working together, try to ease some of the burdens we have in common.

There are very few people today who haven't had at least some connection with Alzheimer's. Nevertheless, a surprising number of those who know something about the disease haven't a clue about what it's like to be a caregiver for someone who has it. In many ways, the Alzheimer's caregiver's job is doomed to failure. Going into the job, she knows she will fail. She will never be able to nurse her patient back to health; he will continue to get worse no matter what she does. "It's a challenging job", we're told, and they're certainly right about that. But "challenging" really means, "This is an extremely difficult job, but you can accomplish it if you're willing to work hard enough". It also implies that, if you can't do it, you've somehow come up short. No wonder we are stressed.

There is no question that being a caregiver for someone with Alzheimer's changes your life. It plays a dominant role in shaping our whole outlook on life. When it happened to us, after many years of successful marriage, it was particularly devastating, because we'd always thought of our lives together as one comfortable unit. We were approaching the aging process with equanimity, and talking about contentedly growing old together. We understood each other so well that we were sure we'd be fine. When Alzheimer's pillaged our lives, it destroyed that illusion and we were left to find our way forward the best way we could.

These caregiving years have forced me to be introspective about our strengths and weaknesses and the nature of our relationship. Has this self-analysis been useful? Yes, I think so. Examining your lives together from a different vantage point is much like standing in front of a complicated painting, attempting to understand what the artist is trying to tell you. At first, you notice only the obvious things, the colors, familiar objects, and maybe the way it makes you feel. But the longer you look, the more you see. Eventually you discover there's a lot more going on here than you thought. You begin to see things you overlooked before, and start to think about how they might contribute to a much broader understanding of what makes up the whole. If you can do this, if you can figure out what it was that made your marriage work all these years, through good times and bad, there's a good chance it will help you see more clearly what strengths you have to work with during this endurance trial called Alzheimer's. And maybe, just maybe, it will make your life and the things you want to accomplish, a little less difficult.

Those of us who have been taking the Alzheimer's journey for a long time now, sometimes feel that we've headed into a long, dark, one-way tunnel. Unfortunately the only light at the end of this tunnel is far behind us. There will be no happy ending.

I think we can all agree that this job is especially daunting, because there's no way to prepare for it. We learn as we go along. We face countless opportunities to make the wrong choice, but we'll never know what the right choice might have been, or even if there was one. And, as if that isn't enough to bear, we watch our loved one gradually slip away from us, in spite of all our efforts. It's unbelievably frustrating. It's not surprising that we begin to feel as if we're being tested, and to fear we will ultimately fail. This is the time when we need all the support we can get. Many have taken this journey already, others are doing it now, and many more will face it in the future. Yes, we understand that. But who will tell us what we need to do now?

One thing we can do is to learn from those who have already been through it, by asking questions and comparing our experiences with theirs. We need to let down our guard long enough to say,

"Help me! I'm not sure how much longer I can do this."

We need to stop thinking that maybe we're just being overly dramatic; that our experience isn't really as awful as we think it is, when we try to tell others about the hell we're going through. We need to summon up the courage to keep telling our story. Because someday there will be someone who listens. Someone who says,

"Yes, I believe what you're going through is truly awful. I understand what you're telling me, and it must be very hard for both of you. Would it help you if we talked about it?"

Once we've admitted that we can't fill the job of caregiver without help, we'll have started to free our minds of the notion that we're expected to do it alone. Only then will we be ready to go out and find the help we need.

CODA

The last time I saw my father, he had finally gone to live in a nursing home. I'm not sure he remembered me, but he smiled and nodded as if he did. After seeing him so obviously relaxed and comfortable in this setting, I felt relief for both my parents. After waiting for what we had all thought was much too long, Mother had finally agreed to an arrangement that she could accept. She missed him terribly, but the constant stress and worry were gone now. I think Dad had finally been able to relax in the nursing home as well as he did, because he'd somehow understood that he would no longer be a burden to Mother. A few months later, he died quietly in his sleep.

For many years after his death, I couldn't bear to hear the Debussy Quartet, but eventually I was able to enjoy it again. Hearing that familiar music today still reminds me of how much I miss Dad. But it also brings back all the special things I remember about him, and the music we enjoyed together.

It's almost unbearable to watch someone you love slowly being taken away from you by dementia. We feel grief and failure when we think of all the years we've spent, trying to save this person we love so much. We've never given up trying, and we've never really stopped hoping. But, back in that place where we put things that are too painful to acknowledge, there's one truth we can no longer avoid. We've known all along that this was one battle we were not going to win.

When I look back over all the years I've been with Chuck, I recall so many things I'm grateful for. We've had a magnificent life together; doing almost all of the things we wanted to do. When Alzheimer's has finally finished with us, I will grieve, as I've been doing for a long time now. But all those memories we stored up over the years are too good to forget. I will try to be the one who remembers them for both of us.

ACKNOWLEDGEMENTS

I'd like to thank the following people for the part they've played in making this book a reality:

My family, for their steadfast support and acknowledgement of the difficulties I faced.

Chuck's family, for their understanding and help during times that were hard for all of us.

Linda Dacey, and her staff, whose ongoing support made it possible for me to continue when I wasn't sure I could.

All the staff at "Harris", for their skill, empathy, and thoughtful care at all times.

My wonderful friends, who helped me to understand that I needed to talk, and who listened to me patiently while I did.

Our group, *The Six*, for the opportunity to talk about common problems within a comfortable environment.

All the people who shared their stories with me and those who encouraged me to write about my own.

Dr. Robert Santulli, who supported my effort to write about Alzheimer's caregivers, and who graciously agreed to write the foreword to this book.

Made in the USA
Columbia, SC
29 September 2019